The Frugal Diet

By Michael J. Schiemer B.S. CSCS CPT

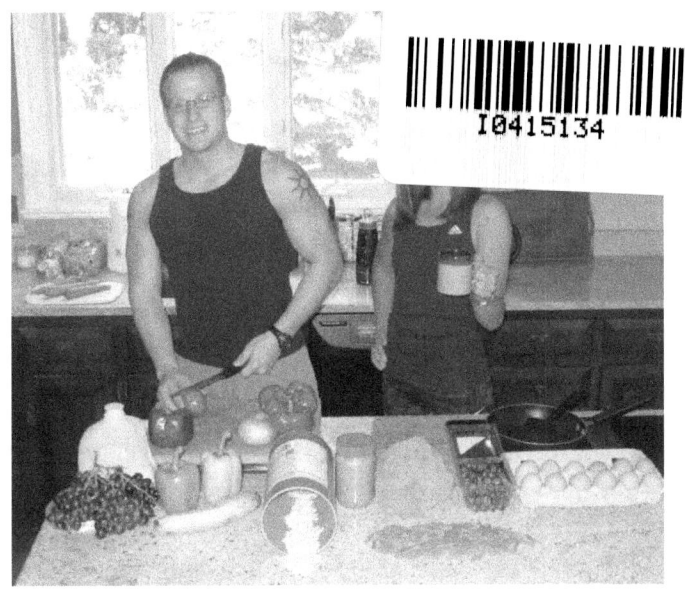

I0415134

Edited By Amanda Baldi and Michael J. Schiemer

Pictured On Cover: Michael J. Schiemer and Julie Zaia

Photographers: Peter Swiniarski, Robert Thomson, David A. Schiemer, Michael J. Schiemer

The Frugal Diet Challenge

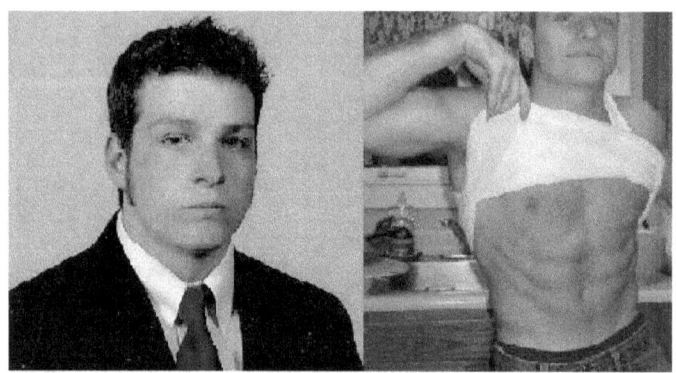

My Frugal Diet Success Story: This Could Be You!

I wrote this book to help everyday people lose weight, improve their fitness level, and save money in both the short term and long term. While improving your daily nutrition and exercise is a lifetime commitment, I encourage you all to take The Frugal Diet 90 Day Challenge to challenge you to improve your health and bank account. After reading this book, use it as a reference to improve your food choices, eating strategies, and purchasing power. Write what you used to weight, eat, and spend before you read this book and then keep track of that information over the next 90 days. After taking the 90 Day Challenge along with the included Frugal Workout, The Complete Frugal Workout, or another workout regimen, compare your numbers and see how you have improved physically and financially! The three people with the best Frugal Diet 90 Day Challenge results will win fantastic prizes! Here is what you have to do:

Step 1: Write down your food, weight, and purchasing information from before you read this book. Take pictures of yourself and your food receipts for a better chance of winning. Fill out the Goal Sheet found later in this book.

Step 2: Implement the strategies, foods, and workouts from this book into your fitness regimen.

Step 3: Use the pages in this book to keep records of your progress. More weekly and daily journal pages can be downloaded from www.resultsprivatefitness.com/thefrugaldiet.html

Step 4: Submit your success story, pictures, and information to Michael J. Schiemer via mikeschiemer@gmail.com by April 30, 2011 to be considered for winning the grand prize! Tell the world how The Frugal Diet helped changed your life for the better!

<u>Contest Prizes:</u>

1st Place: -$100 Visa Gift Card
         -1 Free Year of Online Personal Training
         -Free Frugal Diet T-shirt

2nd Place: -$50 Visa Gift Card
         -3 Free Months of Online Personal Training
         -Free Frugal Diet T-shirt

3rd Place: -$25 Visa Gift Card
         -1 Free Month of Online Personal Training
         -Free Frugal Diet T-shirt

Contest Terms and Conditions:

**Download Your Fitness Journal and Goal Sheets Free at
www.resultsprivatefitness.com/thefrugaldiet.html**

Paperbacks By Michael J. Schiemer

- The Frugal Diet
- The Frugal Workout (Coming In 2011)

E-Books By Michael J. Schiemer
Download To Your Computer or Phone

- The Frugal Workout
- The Frugal Diet
- The Ultimate Nutrition Guide
- The Ultimate Guide To A Healthy Spine
- The Ultimate Guide To Healthy Shoulders

Coming Soon:
- The Ultimate Guide to Toned Abs
- The Ultimate Guide to a Toned Butt
- The Ultimate Guide to Healthy Knees
- The Ultimate Guide to Nutritional Supplements
- The Ultimate Guide to Bench Press
- Strength and Conditioning for Wrestling
- Strength and Conditioning for Hockey
- Strength and Conditioning for Gymnastics
- Strength and Conditioning for Track/Cross Country
- Strength and Conditioning for Football

Blog's Available By Subscription:

- The Ultimate Sports, Science, Health, & Fitness Blog
- The Ultimate Business, Marketing, & Economics Blog
- The Ultimate Lifestyle & Culture Blog
- The Ultimate Pet & Animal Blog

Medical Disclaimer

Michael J. Schiemer is not a physician and this book is not a substitute for medical advice. Consult with a physician before beginning an exercise or nutrition regimen. Products and services offered by Michael J. Schiemer and RESULTS Private Fitness LLC are not intended to cure, prevent, or treat any disease or condition. Michael J. Schiemer and RESULTS Private Fitness LLC are not liable for any harm incurred from product or service use. Exercise always carries an inherent risk. Dietary supplements are not currently regulated by the FDA and may cause harm, side effects, or interactions with certain drugs. Health and fitness advice in this book may be based on personal experiences or publicly available information and should be confirmed with your physician before adding to your regimen.

Legal Disclaimer

Michael J. Schiemer and Results Private Fitness LLC do not officially endorse any specific products, services, companies, or brands. Michael J. Schiemer is not sponsored in any way by any of the products or companies mentioned in this book. All designated / registered trademarks, copyrighted works, product names, company names, or logos contained in this website are the property of their respective owners. Recipes submitted by others to Michael J. Schiemer were stated by contributors as being unique and their intellectual property.

Author's Note:

Advice and recommendations given in this book are from personal experience, experience with thousands of clients, and my specific education. These are merely personal suggestions and should not be used as a nutritional bible or instead of physician recommendations. Results will vary from person to person due to a myriad of factors. Many complicated concepts and scientific topics have been simplified for easier reading. The prices reflected in this book are estimates from personal experience and may vary from city, state, and country. These prices are based in the United States. The suggestions in this book are geared towards the average person trying to improve their health and lose fat unless stated otherwise. If you have a unique medical or nutritional condition, the advice in this book may not be appropriate for you. Ask your physician and/or registered dietitian before starting this program or implementing one of the suggestions included in this book.

This book is dedicated to my family, friends, mentors, and clients who believed in me and pushed me to improve myself and expand my horizons.

Acknowledgements

This book was a labor of love and a really fun experience for me. I've been writing workouts and nutrition plans for people since I was 15 years old and I decided it was time to compile and expand everything I've learned over the years in the fitness industry. There is so much to learn about health, fitness, and nutrition and I love how there are always new developments to keep up with. I've always loved to write but I wouldn't have continued if people didn't encourage me and enjoy my writing. Formally writing and publishing a book was a new experience for me and I had a lot of help with it. First, I'd like to thank my parents and family for their constant support and emphasis on living a healthy lifestyle. They have also put up with my frugal lifestyle for many years!

A big thank you also goes out to my editor and advisor Amanda Baldi for deciding to help me take on this project and having faith that it would be a success. She is a phenomenal writer and editor, any mistakes in this book are solely due to me trying to edit it myself. Thank you to all of my friends that encouraged me and contributed recipes for the book. Another very special thanks also goes out to all of my clients over the years that have worked so hard to improve their health and fitness levels. You all consistently continue to inspire me to keep working hard. You are the best clients in the world and it has been a privilege working with all of you. Don't ever stop in your quest for self-improvement!

Table of Contents

Introduction

Today there is greater need for frugality than ever before. Over the last decade, the economy has been pretty lousy and it has taken quite a toll on a lot of good people. Companies are out of business, jobs are being cut, positions are being outsourced, and people are in major debt. The banks aren't lending as much and people are stuck between a rock and a hard place. For a lot of people, the United States does not seem like the land of good and plenty anymore. The rest of the world's economy isn't looking much better either. Many people are cutting back in all areas and sometimes the first thing to get cut out is their investment in health and fitness. When you cut back on health and fitness, often times you will pay for it in the long run with extra trips to the doctor's office, chiropractor, pharmacist, physical therapist, psychiatrist, and so on. You may even find yourself in major surgery if you ignore your health and wellness long enough. While some individuals are in such dire financial straits that they legitimately can't afford many health and fitness products and services, most people just have the wrong set of priorities. Many people out there would rather keep their HBO subscription or buy the new iPhone than put that money towards a gym membership, professional health services, or healthier food. Money should not be an excuse to compromise your health. This book was written to help those in tight financial situations to improve their health and fitness levels for a price that is affordable to everyone.

There is also an incredible need to improve our society's health and fitness levels. The big trend in the United States is the alarming increase in obesity, adult-onset diabetes, cancer, and heart disease. We have consistently hit record highs in all of these categories over the last decade and there aren't any promising signs of the trend reversing. We've become a "super-sized" culture of big meals, fast food, and unhealthy nutrition. People are always stressed out, on the go, and claim they don't have time to sit down to eat or prepare a healthy meal. Everyone's stress, anxiety, and depression levels are at an all time high. Our nation's health and healthcare are both in major jeopardy. Also, Americans work more hours than every other first world nation and we are a very stressed out society because of it. Everyone is looking for the quick fix to all of these problems but nobody is looking at sound nutrition and scientific evidence. I have been working hard over the last decade as a personal trainer to help educate clients and consumers to improve their health and quality of life with a rational approach. There is much more work to be done before we can all make a major positive change in our culture.

To be honest, the last thing I ever thought I would be writing was a diet book. I'm really not a very big fan of many of the diets and diet books out there. So many of the Atkins and South Beach diets out there are completely impractical for the average person to follow and stick to. Eliminating carbohydrates completely, even for a couple of weeks, can prove disastrous for any person's life and health.

The cleansing diets that are all the rage are also very unhealthy and ridiculous in my opinion as well. Human beings were not meant to live on lemon juice and cayenne pepper for days or weeks at a time! If you have ever tried one of these diets, you definitely know what I'm talking about. Crash dieting or other fad dieting does not work for the majority of people. They are very difficult to stick with and when they stop dieting they are even worse off than before. Dieting is not a quick fix, it is a long term lifestyle change. Then there are the diet books out there that are sponsored by nutritional supplement or food product companies. These "diet books" are nothing more than one big written infomercial on their product and how it can single-handedly help you lose 50 lbs or get you ripped. These have no credibility and simply want to brainwash you into buying their products. The nutritional supplement industry is also infamous for its diet pills that claim to work miracles but instead just deliver jitters, disappointment, and a smaller bank account. I didn't want to write just another generic diet book that took a limited weight loss principle to the extreme. I'm not sponsored or working for any food or nutritional supplement company and therefore I am unbiased.

I've always been a cheapskate, but I've also always been a health nut. Now those two things may seem contradictory at first, but that is why I decided to write this book. Over the years I have had dozens of debates about the expenses of eating healthy and how you either have to decide between being broke and being lean and healthy. Every time the subject comes up, I make a point to disprove this misconception and prevent money from being just another excuse for being unhealthy. This book is meant to finally disprove that theory by educating you on proper eating and purchasing strategies. I decided to appeal to the vast majority of people out there that want a safe, realistic, and effective diet that they can stick to and benefit from in multiple ways. I also wanted to create a diet that people could afford to continue financially without expensive foods and supplements. There are hundreds of diet books out there and you might think they are all the same, but this may be the most practical one out there.

I am so confident that The Frugal Diet and Frugal Workout will work for you, that I want you to take The Frugal Diet 90 Day Challenge for weight loss and fitness! As you read this book, begin charting your progress in weight, fitness regimen, food bill, and eating habits. After 90 days you should see a significant improvement and if you submit your success story, you can win great prizes! I sincerely hope it helps you to improve the ways that you eat, exercise, and purchase food. I hope this book not only improves your health and fitness, but also pays for itself the first time you go to the grocery store! Over the years I have seen it work wonders for myself and hundreds of my friends, family, and personal training clients. So who said eating healthy had to be expensive? Enjoy the book and stay healthy!

-Michael J. Schiemer

I

The Frugal Life
"The Cheap, The Bad, and The Ugly"

Initially you may be skeptical that you can eat healthier and lose weight on a tight budget. You will be proven wrong. Eating frugally is a science and I will go into every aspect of it in great detail. The first thing I must do is prove my cheapskate credentials to you. These following true stories will give you an insight into my frugal world. I will first prove to you that I am the absolute authority on being cheap. Then I will prove to you that I am the absolute authority on health and fitness. Then I will tie it all together and teach you how to integrate the two successfully for healthy weight loss and savings. Before we get into how to correctly eat inexpensively, first let's take a quick snapshot of my glamorous frugal life so far.

My frugal credentials are very strong and comprehensive. Ever since I was a young lad I would hoard pennies and small amounts of money like they were hundred dollar bills. I was always one to save money instead of spend it and I always tried to get what I wanted for free if possible. I became famous for my cheapness when I began playing paintball with my friends in middle school. Not only did I buy the cheapest gun possible (The Spyder Compact) and the cheapest paintballs (32 Degrees), but I would infamously run out of paintballs and pick stray ones off the ground to use as ammunition. It didn't matter to me that half of the paintballs were old, dented, and clogged the chamber of my gun. It beat buying more and spending actual money. On other outings, sometimes I would "forget my wallet" and somebody else would have to pay for me. Sometimes they also forgot to ask me to pay them back and I didn't remind them. In return, my friends and roommates would give me a hard time and throw pennies on the floor or down the hall for me to retrieve. I gladly did. What else would you expect from a guy that kept 200 unwashed cans and bottles in his dorm for over a month just to recycle them for less than $10? Some of those were picked out of trash cans too. Sure I did some of it for the environment or a charity, but I also did some of it for the precious nickel redemptions.

Some of the most extreme cases of being a cheapskate took the form of "borrowing" toilet paper from public bathrooms and using the rolls in my own dorm room. Sometimes I would even take rolls that were half used already! This wasn't even double-ply, this was the thinnest and least comfortable toilet paper ever invented. The places I got this toilet from had a budget almost as frugal as my own. I did all of this just to save $1 a roll or less. I could have gone to the store and gotten a comfortable and high quality brand for a few bucks but instead I would smuggle out the goods like they were worth their weight in gold.

My relationships have provided excellent examples of my frugality. With each girlfriend I would initially spend a decent amount of money on dates. Then like clockwork I would eventually get financially depleted and use money as an excuse to stay in. That meant my girlfriends had two choices, either stay in or pay for me. Often times they started paying for me, and needless to say the relationships didn't last much longer beyond that point. On a few occasions, I would suggest going out to a specific restaurant for a date night. They would be impressed I was taking them out until the bill came and I pulled out my gift card to that specific restaurant. If I had a restaurant gift card, that was definitely where we were going out to eat! My poor ex-girlfriends had to deal with a lot of this nonsense. Also the fact that I've fervently argued the merits of cubic zirconia over diamonds hasn't helped either. After hearing that little tidbit, they rightfully lost what little respect and interest in me that they may have had. Needless to say, I am single now and will most likely continue to be unless I win the lottery. Any woman claiming that money isn't important should try dating me for a few months! That might change their tune.

I try to take some pride in my personal appearance but not at the cost of an arm and a leg. I am proud to say that I don't own one pair of pants of any type that cost over $20 and I only own about four shirts that cost more than that. Even my suits cost about $150 a piece which isn't too bad. I frequent Wal-Mart for a lot of my clothing and accessories, occasionally resorting to the Wal-Mart clearance racks for even better values. A lot of my dress shoes and boots cost me about $15 at Payless Shoes and nobody can tell the difference. That is until I brag about it and induce gratuitous laughter or eye-rolling. I used to have a couple $300 watches that were given as gifts from family but they both broke so I decided no more expensive jewelry. The variety of $8 watches I've bought from Wal-Mart are the best watches I've ever owned and the ones that have gotten me the most compliments. If one of them breaks, or even runs out of batteries for that matter, I can just toss it and buy a new one! I'm also not ashamed to say that I own a few ties from the Salvation Army that cost me 50 cents or less per tie. The Dollar Tree has provided me with so many 3-packs of socks for one dollar that I could probably go a year without doing laundry. If I absolutely can't find what I'm looking for at all these low cost venues, I will visit Kohls or a Marshalls for slightly more expensive options. On other days, I find exactly what I am looking for in the gym or school Lost and Found box. Don't worry I wash it all!

On the topic of appearances, I also cringe at the thought of paying a lot of money for a haircut. I don't know how so many women (and some men) consistently pay up to $100 or more for getting their hair done. In the past I have gone many months without getting a haircut, to the point of nearly owning my very own mullet. With the help of an old Boston Red Sox hat I used to wear everyday, I think I went 8 months once without getting a haircut just to save money. I've also gone the opposite way and buzzed my head which is another free alternative. I have a little bit of a receding hair line and I'm naturally pretty pale, so I didn't look very good with a buzz cut. The price was right though so I did it about half a dozen times. Now I have graduated to getting my hair cut every month but at a reasonably priced place like Supercuts. Can't beat a haircut for $15.

While my dream car is a Mercedes roadster convertible, my actual car is a Hyundai Accent. While it is a decent car, it's pretty much the opposite of a Mercedes. Not only is it cheap to begin with, but it doesn't have any power locks, windows, or air conditioning because they cost too much extra. At the time I bought the car, I figured all of those power options and air conditioning were just more things that could break and cost me more money in repairs. Plus, rolling down the windows (literally) is like free air conditioning! Unfortunately that hypothesis was proven false on a 95 degree day when I was stuck in traffic. Without air conditioning in my car I guess I won't be moving to the deep south anytime soon. It is great on gas though, getting

36 miles per gallon on the highway! I even put larger wheels on it, a K&N high flow air filter, and consistently add fuel injector cleaners to keep the gas mileage up even higher. Mercedes just can't beat the free roadside assistance and 10 year/100,000 mile warranty!

Even my pet choice is affected by my frugal lifestyle! I have grown up with dogs all my life and I am definitely a "dog person". Surprisingly though I don't currently have a dog, I have a cat as my only pet. One of my personal training clients had found the stray cat in her yard and asked me if I wanted it. I said sure. Luckily my new cat Chewie acts more like a dog than a cat and has been a wonderful pet. Cats are obviously much lower maintenance and less expensive than dogs so she fits in better with my frugal lifestyle. Since I don't have my own dog, I decided to start a side business (Responsible Pet Care) doing dog walking and pet care. Not only would I be able to spend time with some great dogs without the expense, but I could get paid for it on top of that! While it isn't the same as having your own dog, it is good enough for me at this point and definitely a better option for my bank account.

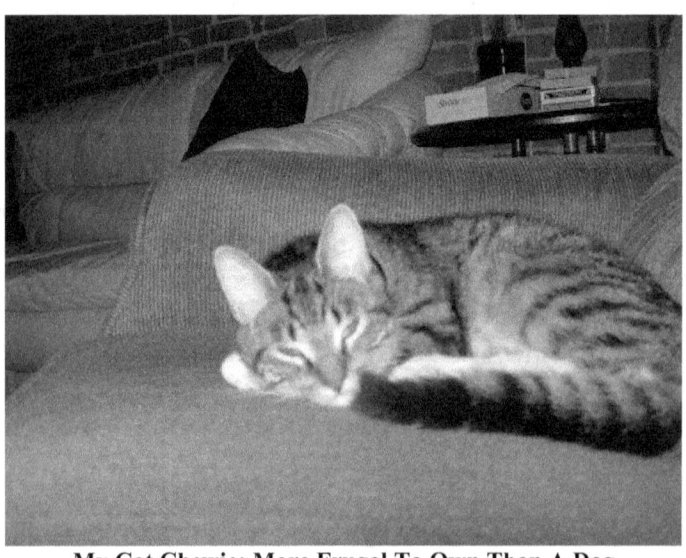

My Cat Chewie: More Frugal To Own Than A Dog

Even my businesses are a reflection of my frugal state of mind. My personal training business, for instance, has been tailored to be financially feasible for nearly all walks of life. Traditionally, personal training is considered an expensive luxury service that only wealthy people could enjoy, but I have worked to break that tradition. I offer personal training to clients at a guaranteed lowest price in the industry and allowed many individuals a valuable opportunity that they normally would not have had to improve their wellness. I've trained dozens of clients over the years that were lower class, out of a job, or just graduating from college with massive student loans. I also offer many different ways for my clients to earn or win free personal training sessions for hard work, advertising for me, referrals, and special offers. I personally enjoy getting top value for my money and believe others should as well.

My internet marketing consulting business, RESULTS Business Solutions, is also about drastically reducing my clients' marketing budgets through web, email, and social media advertising campaigns. This strategy is often low in cost, high in value, and sometimes even free on top of my consulting rates. While companies can spend thousands of dollars on websites, business listings, and internet advertising, I show businesses how to utilize as many low cost or free services as possible to get the same benefits. RESULTS Business Solutions also guarantees the lowest prices in the industry to make it available to any business looking to improve their marketing and profit margins. These methods also help to conserve paper and energy waste and help companies go green.

I advertise both of my businesses the cheapest and more efficient possible ways. I use a myriad of free social media sites to get tons of traffic to my websites and listings. I also produce all of my unique content including writing, videos, and products. My websites are relatively inexpensive each month and I designed every single aspect of them myself so I didn't have to pay anyone else. I put tacky but effective car door magnets, window decals, and bumper stickers all over my car since I drive around so much and after the initial small cost, it is free advertising. The only thing I've ever really spent any money on for advertising is small amounts for business cards and slightly more for client t-shirts. I even make deals with other small businesses to exchange advertising or services for more advertising. Over the years I've also done my fair share of grassroots marketing such as leaving my business cards and flyers on car windshield wipers, in bank ATM kiosks, and all over community boards. At a young age I even got in trouble for dropping off flyers into neighbors mailboxes. Apparently it's illegal to bypass the post office, oh well live and learn. Overall I get excellent returns on my small marketing investments so why pay more for traditional advertising?

Finally, my past nutrition has been greatly influenced by cost. I warn you that the following are not healthy examples of how to eat to save money. These tales are from the years before I came up with The Frugal Diet and the results were not pretty. Kids, don't try this at home. Let's see, where to begin. I've purchased Beef Jerky at the Dollar Store and the nutritional label assured me it was "Inspected by the Brazilian Government". No offense to the Brazilian Government, but that claim didn't exactly make me feel very secure about what I was eating. It also vaguely says the meat was "inspected" but does not specifically say it was "approved". Beef jerky is not the worst thing you can eat (nearly fat free and no carbohydrates) but it does have a large amount of sodium nitrites for flavor and preservative. These sodium nitrites have been classified as carcinogens (cancer-causing) and should be avoided in significant amounts. On another occasion I also purchased a 4 pound generic tub of chocolate whey protein for $8 because it was already expired. It was by far the worst tasting protein powder that I've ever had but I consumed every scoop of that tub over the next several months. By the time I was done with it, I think the protein had been expired for about a year. Are you convinced of my frugality yet? Unfortunately, I'm just getting started.

The madness doesn't end there. Freshman year of college I ate horribly, indulging on cocoa puffs, hot chocolate, pizza, beer, and ramen noodles nearly everyday. If it was free or dirt cheap I would eat or drink it. In college I also used to consistently go to the local Panera Bread to run in, raid the free bread sample bowl, and run out. If I was actually staying in to eat, I would also fill up a free water cup with as much skim milk as possible from the coffee station. If I was lucky, I'd even get to eat the leftovers or chips from the friends that I came with. On the few occasions that I caught a Red Sox game at Fenway Park, I'd always bring in food and water so I wouldn't have to pay $7 per item in the ballpark. When I went to Chile's, I always ordered Endless Tostado Chips because they only cost $2 and came with unlimited salsa and refills. I would eat about a bowl or two and call it a meal. Of course, I would also order water at no charge for my trademark beverage. Bertuccis was even better because I just had plenty of rolls with butter or oil for free. Let's just say the waitresses weren't too fond of me and I didn't put anybody through college with my tips. It must have been quite embarrassing to go out to eat with me. You might also wonder who gets up at 5 am to get free coffee at McDonalds. I hated waking up early but I did it on a few occasions just for free caffeine. Free condiments were always appealing to me as well. On more than one occasion I strolled into a Starbucks or Dunkin Donuts and grabbed massive amounts of Splenda, Sweet and Low, Equal, regular Sugar, Sugar in the Raw, and napkins for my apartment. If I went out to breakfast, I would often take a few of their little containers of syrup, jelly, jam, or butter for myself as well. On the few occasions I went to weddings, I was that guy that stands next to the shrimp all night stuffing his face. Maybe that is why I haven't been invited to many weddings. When I traveled to Montreal with several friends, I lived each time on 99 cent pizza slices, a jar of peanut butter, and $1 baguettes (not counting the alcohol). When the Red Bull girls came to my college on a slow day to give out free samples, I convinced them to give me the rest of their samples. I told them it would be less work for them if they gave me 20 free red bulls and I gave them out to my friends. Of course I ended up keeping most of them for myself.

When it came to drinking alcohol, I was never as crazy as most of my friends. I did partake in some partying though over the years. Alcohol and partying cost money though so I was always looking for ways to cut back. I would purchase the cheapest bottom shelf vodka possible, the kind that cost $9 for a handle and smelled/tasted like rubbing alcohol. I would mix it with diet store brand soda and enjoy the worst tasting mixed drink every created. For beer, I would also buy the cheapest possible brand, often being Busch Light or Milwaukee's Best by the 30 rack. Sure it tasted like tainted tap water, but it was still technically beer. I even famously drank Budweisers that were 4 years old from a friend's basement and other Budweisers that had been in my car's trunk for weeks. Needless to say, that beer didn't sit too well. As you can imagine, I also mooched a lot of beers as well when I could.

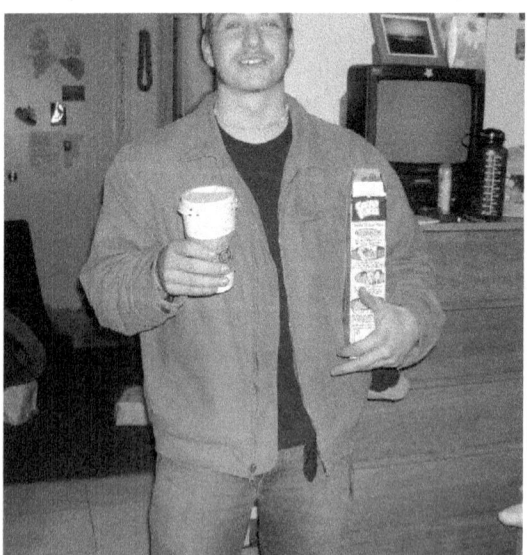

**Freshman Year of College Eating Cocoa Puffs
And Drinking Hot Chocolate**

When it came to wine I purchased only the finest boxes of Franzia. At 5 liters for $5-10, you just couldn't go wrong. Occasionally I would go a little classier and buy some Wal-Mart Wine for $3 a bottle in New Hampshire. For champagne, there was nothing better than $5 bottles of Andre. Many a New Year's party had me showing up with nothing but 2 bottles of Andre for myself. The savings didn't end there either. If I went to bars I probably had previously engaged in the tradition known as "pre-gaming". If you don't know, this is when you drink a lot of alcohol before you go out to the bars or party. By the time you got to the bar or party, you would be pretty intoxicated and only have to buy 1 or 2 drinks at their high prices. Needless to say, I didn't go to a lot of classy bars or even bars or clubs with covers. When I was finally at the bar, I would often order their drink specials or the cheapest beer they had on tap. I'm pretty sure a few times I also snuck into the bar with a flask or a few pocket beers so I didn't have to order many or any drinks.

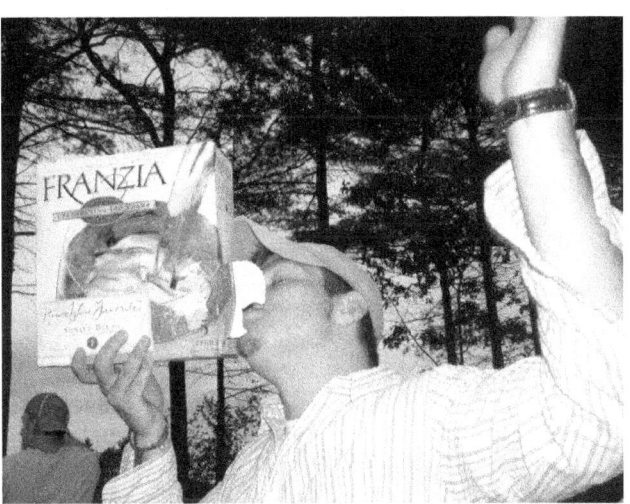
Kids Don't Try This At Home

When I got my first real apartment and had to pay for utilities, I did everything I could to minimize costs. I survived until the end of November before turning on the heat for the first time and instead just wore more clothing and slept with an extra blanket. This was north of Boston mind you. I also switched all of my lights to LEDs since they required 90% less electricity than normal light bulbs. It didn't matter that I couldn't see very well, darkness was free! If I needed extra light, I would just light a few candles I got at the local dollar store. One time I bought an old $40 recliner at the Salvation Army a quarter mile down the street from me and I didn't want to pay someone to deliver it to my apartment. Why should I pay $25 to have it shipped down the street when I could walk it down the street on top of my head? It didn't matter that it was a 95 degree day and I was dehydrated. My feat of strength and stupidity turned a lot of heads as I walked down the main street of Haverhill Massachusetts with a huge recliner on my head. It almost killed me, but I walked that recliner all the way down the street and up into my apartment. I ended up cutting myself on the rusty metal underneath the chair and had to pay $100 for a tetanus shot, but I was due for a new one anyways. I still have that recliner to this very day at least. On various occasions I would often think about saving rent money by living out of a van and joining a 24 hour fitness club to use the locker rooms. I've never actually taken any steps to follow through on this pipe dream but every time I write out my rent check it does seem rather tempting.

Free samples may be my two favorite words in the entire world. I have taken the concept of free samples to the absolute extreme on many an occasion. I will take free samples of things I don't even like and stock up on them just because they are free. I used to grab free books from schools, libraries, businesses, and our town's swap shop and either educate myself with them or sell them on e-store sites. At one point I had about 2,000 books in stock and an overall revenue of about $12,000 from selling stuff I got mostly for free! Free samples of energy drinks, moisturizers, keychains, flashlights, deodorant spray, and anything else you can think of made me very happy indeed! I like to workout at home but when I do go to a gym I make sure to get a complimentary weekly gym pass to try it out. In college one year, I got so many samples of free safety razors and shaving cream that I'm still using them to this very day. I don't have a lot of facial hair so all of the samples I got may end up lasting me for the rest of my life. I can only hope. I even got in trouble a few times for taking too many free samples that were meant "only for customers" from a place I worked at. Needless to say, a lot of friends and family (even girlfriends) have gotten some of the free samples I've procured as birthday and Christmas present. Hey, it's the thought that counts!

Now I know what you're thinking. What does any of this have to do with eating healthy? So far I've merely mentioned my cheap exploits and many unhealthy examples of how to save money. I obviously don't endorse eating and living like I did, but so far this is just a backdrop on how to be innovative to save money. When you apply these strategies to eating for weight loss and general health, you can reap many benefits. Now that you've read the bad and the ugly, read on to learn the positive methods of eating cheaply that I actually recommend.

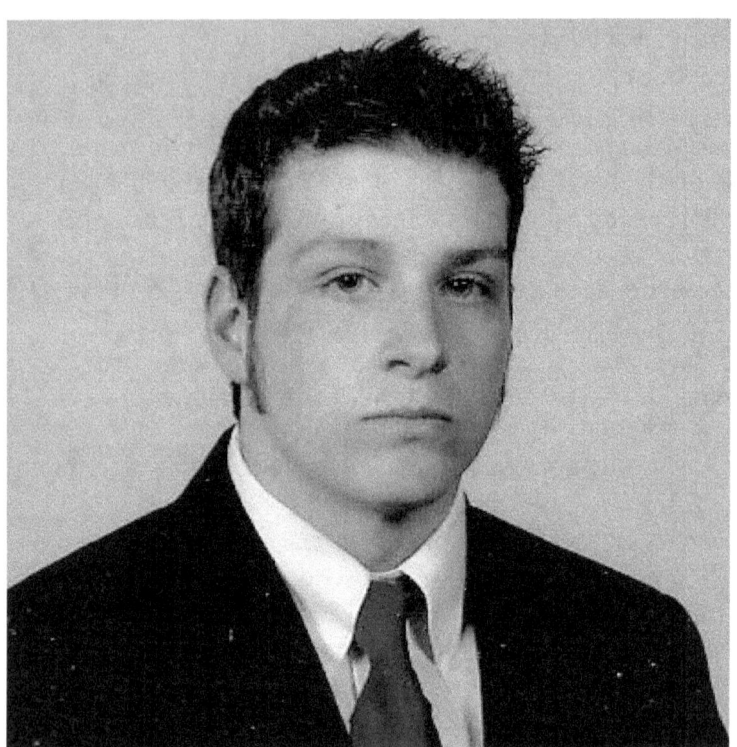

The Face of an Unhealthy Freshman Cheapskate (Pre-Frugal Diet)

II

The Frugal Inspiration
"The Good"

Now here is where the healthy part of being frugal comes in. After screwing around a bit my first few months of college, I became very busy and disciplined. I started working long hours at the college gym, getting excellent grades as an exercise physiology major, and building up my personal training clientele. I continued being cheap because I was making low wages and also worried about paying off my impending student loans. I decided that I needed to start focusing on improving my health and fitness for optimal performance in all of my endeavors. That meant I would need to start eating more for function and not for taste. I also had to get the most out of all of my food purchases or in essence I'd be wasting money. I would go to the Merrimack College cafeteria and really try to make the most out of my meal plan of 13 meals per week. That meant I could eat less than 2 meals a day on average, including weekends. For somebody that worked out five times a week and was trying to put on muscle, that wasn't very much. I knew I couldn't go in and eat all the pizza, fried chicken, and stale desserts they served every day. I knew if I did that, I would be hungry again within an hour and I would have low energy all day. I switched to eating wheat toast and peanut butter or turkey with spicy mustard. I ate a lot of granola, tuna, and eggs as well. I'd only drink skim milk, black coffee, and tea instead of three glasses of soda or fake fruit juice like my peers. There certainly weren't many other students in the cafeteria that ate this way. I saw how everybody else ate at the cafeteria and immediately discovered why so many college students put on the dreaded "Freshman 15".

I would also supplement my meal plan with other cheap, versatile, and healthy foods to help keep me going throughout the day. I would always have at least a gallon of skim milk on hand and a tub of protein powder for workouts and snacks. In my backpack I would always have a bag of Kashi cereal, a container of almonds, and a jar of sunflower seed kernels. I always carried around plenty of water as well to keep hydrated and avoid cravings for junk food. I had so many snacks on hand that my friends would joke that I had a food pantry in my backpack and in the passenger seat of my car. I would always have a jar of peanut butter in my dorm room if needed. Instead of eating the traditional American three big meals per day, I learned to graze on healthy food every couple of hours to keep my metabolism up and bodyfat down. I even competed in my first natural bodybuilding competitions junior year of college.

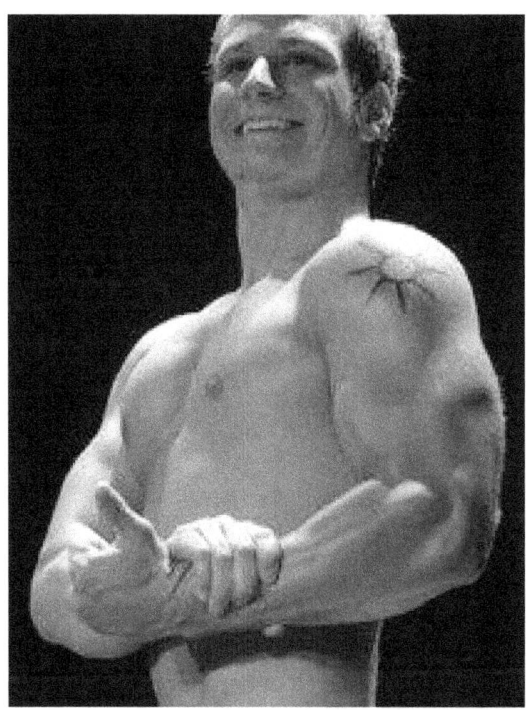

My First Natural Bodybuilding Competition
(Original Photo by Todd Ganci)

When senior year came along and I finally had a kitchen. I dropped my meal plan and ended up saving about $1,000 buying and cooking my own meals instead. I also dropped some serious bodyfat that year. I still kept the staples of skim milk, protein powder, peanut butter, almonds, sunflower seed kernels, Kashi, and tea but I began to add in more complete meals. I started grilling up chicken breasts, omelettes, making whole grain pasta, making whole grain pancakes, and even cooking healthy pizzas. I would also mooch off of my friends that still had meal plans and extra meals so I could get free healthy food from the college cafeteria. At the supermarket I realized there were plenty of other healthy foods that I could purchase very cheaply including tuna, brown rice, vegetables, whole grain toast/bagels/English muffins, canola oil, flaxseeds, and more. I also bought boxes in bulk of green tea and tried to drink a cup or two per day for the extra antioxidants and metabolism boost. With the addition of healthier food and more tea in my diet, I stopped getting the chronic sinus infections that had plagued me every winter of my life. I still partied with friends here and there but I drank less often, less alcohol, and went out to eat less often. By the end of my senior year of college, I had made many improvements in the nutrition department on my limited budget and it was significantly improving my health and physique. Even though I ate and worked out to maintain or gain weight, I got down to about 8% bodyfat with my new nutrition plan and workout regimen. By the time I received my degree in exercise physiology, graduating with honors, I was in excellent shape and utilizing my Frugal Diet plan for all it was worth. I even had saved enough money to pay off all of my student loans with one check! It all finally clicked and I knew there was something to this frugal fitness strategy. I've been utilizing The Frugal Diet for years now and I've been able to keep my muscle mass up, bodyfat down, and health very good. Over the years I've been encouraging others to do the same and reap the health and money-saving benefits that I have been enjoying.

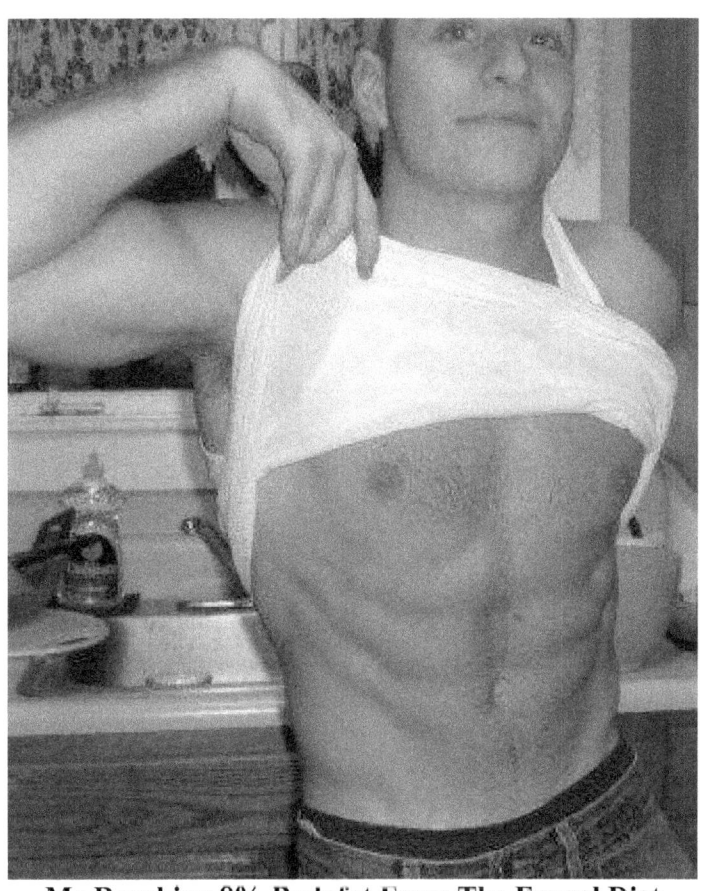

Me Reaching 8% Bodyfat From The Frugal Diet

III

Frugal Tips

There are a plethora of helpful tips to know when it comes to getting the best nutrition for your dollar. Some of these tips may be common sense to you but some of them will be new. Either way, it is still helpful to see them and have them in the back of your head next time you are out to eat or at the grocery store. Every little bit helps to add up to big savings and improvements in weight and physique. It may take a little while for all these improvements to accumulate but they will ultimately benefit you in many ways. Read on and implement as many of these frugal tips as possible.

Learn Frugal-nomics

This is obviously just a term I made up but the more basic principles of economics you understand, the easier it is for you to reap the benefits and save money on your food products. If there is a high supply of healthy food, the price may be lower. If there is a low demand for a healthy food, the price may also be lower. If a merchant or company can produce a healthy product for less money or increase their efficiency, a lower price may be reflected. Companies that don't have to spend as much marketing their products can afford to sell their products for less money. If there are multiple companies trying to sell a similar health food product, the prices may be driven down by competition. When you purchase a food item you need to do at least a quick cost-benefit analysis to determine whether the product is a smart choice. Determine ahead of time what you are trying to achieve with your food choices and try and satisfy those goals as cheaply as possible. These are all very simple and common situations that you need to evaluate and benefit from.

Learn To Read Food Labels

This might be the most crucial tip for eating healthier and saving money. If you don't know how to effectively read the nutritional labels on foods, you are just guessing or poking around in the dark. You need to know the significance of the serving sizes, calorie content, types of fat, types of carbohydrates, amount of protein, and various other nutrients. You ideally want to purchase foods with minimal or no saturated fat, cholesterol, and sugars. You normally want to go for foods with high amounts of fiber, protein, and micronutrients such as vitamins and minerals. Generally, the fewer ingredients that are listed, the better. If the ingredients list reads like a chemistry textbook, chances are the food is not very natural and may have a lot of junk in it that you don't want to put into your body. Overall, if you don't know how to read nutritional labels, how will you figure out how to find healthy foods at low prices? This especially comes in handy when you are comparing two similar products so you can purchase the cheaper one. Be sure to read the section "How To Read A Food Label" in the next chapter.

Buy In Bulk

One of the best ways to ensure that you are getting a good price on food is to purchase it in bulk. Obviously the company producing it saves on packaging and you get a discount for the large volume. If there is a food or product that you know you will be consuming a lot of for a long time, purchase it in the largest amounts possible. You of course need to take into consideration if and when the good expires but for many goods that will not be an issue. A lot of companies out there such as BJ's and Costco offer very large amounts of food and supplements for very low prices. In the case of nutritional supplements, if you purchase very large amounts you may be able to get them at wholesale prices. Some excellent items to buy in bulk include whole grain pasta, brown rice, peanuts, peanut butter, almonds, tuna, sunflower seeds, whole grain cereals, coffee, tea, diet soda, and protein powder. Pretty much anything that doesn't spoil quickly is fine to buy in bulk. You can also buy relatively large amounts of chicken breasts, grill them all up at once, and then eat them throughout the week.

Shop At Discount Stores

As I mentioned in the first chapter, I am a huge fan of discount stores such as Wal-Mart, Dollar Tree, BJ's, Costco, Market Basket, etc for food purchases. Sure, the service and atmosphere is not always as nice as the more expensive stores, but the product is there and it is cheap. You don't need to go to Whole Foods for an apple when you can buy the same one ten times cheaper at another store. Do you want to pay for ambiance or do you want to pay for food that can help you get in better shape? Purchasing food at a cheaper store does not necessarily mean you will get a lower quality product. Often times, you will be purchasing the same exact product for a lower price at these discount stores. When it comes to fresh meat and produce, you may want to look to a farmer's market instead or just make sure the product you are purchasing is fresh and high quality. Farmer's markets usually get their food locally while big discount stores may import their meat and produce from around the globe.

Buy Generic

Generic or store brand food products are often another great way to save a lot of cash. These companies save money with minimal or no advertising or by producing it in their own factories and the savings are passed to the consumer. Often times, the store brand is the exact same product or has the exact same ingredients as the brand name. The best way to ensure that you are getting the same high quality product is to hold up both products next to each other and read the nutritional information and ingredients. Compare them both and make sure that they match up evenly. I've even found many generic products that I like better than the original so it is a win-win situation.

Skip The Organic Foods

You may be very surprised to see this one on my list of frugal nutrition tips but for the most part it is true. Organic foods are not necessarily better than their "inorganic" counterparts. Organic foods are supposed to be defined as food that is uncorrupted by unnatural food additives, genetic engineering, or pesticides. Organic is often sometimes just a word on the food label or a marketing strategy companies use to increase prices and sales. It is now a loosely defined marketing buzz word right now that shouldn't make or break all of your food purchasing decisions. If you can get organic foods for a cheap price (think Trader Joe's), then by all means go for it. If your requirement is to purchase nothing but organic products, you will end up spending a fortune and not necessarily being any healthier or leaner for it. In my opinion, organic foods are nice but not at the expense of your whole paycheck.

Minimize Alcohol

When it comes to drinking alcohol, the less you drink the better. Ideally you do not want to drink any alcohol because it is simply an empty source of calories, liver damage, and brain damage. Since most people don't want to quit drinking completely, here are a few methods to drink "healthier" and for a lower cost. Before you drink, make sure you take in plenty of water and healthy food. This will ensure that you are hydrated, the alcohol won't hit your system all at once, and you will feel fuller and therefore less likely to drink to excess. Alcohol is a diuretic which means that it will dehydrate you significantly. While you are drinking, continue to take breaks and drink water to help you stay hydrated and keep your stomach's pH level more balanced. Switch from soda to generic diet soda to save money and significantly reduce your sugar and calories. Cheap light beer will also save you calories and money but that doesn't mean you have permission to drink twice as much. Try to take advantage of the beer specials or cheap drafts if possible to keep the cost down, especially if they include light beer. Try to keep moving to burn calories and avoid sitting for long periods of time. Finally, rehydrate with water or a diluted sports drink before going to sleep.

Only Bring (Minimal) Cash Out To Bars

This goes along with the previous tip of minimizing alcohol intake. If you know you are going out to a bar (or a wedding with a cash bar), don't bring your credit or debit cards with you! Only bring a small amount of cash with you out to the bars so that there is a much smaller chance that you will spend and drink an exorbitant amount. If you only have $20 to spend, you probably won't be able to drink 8 or 10 beers and you will be all the better for that. I guess you also might need to have a little cab fare on you as well but you can't spend that on booze instead. Not only will this tip help your midsection and bank account, it will also eliminate any risk that you will lose or get your credit cards stolen.. I've known people that have lost their credit cards at bars and ended up with final tabs of over $1,000 from someone who had picked it up and started using it as their own. Dealing with credit card companies and banks to rectify a situation such as this isn't fun or frugal!

Educate Yourself on Nutrition

This crucial tip goes along with the first one of learning to read nutritional labels on foods. This book is an excellent guide to improving your health and nutrition so you are already ahead of the game. That being said, the more legitimate research you do on health and nutrition the better off you will be. Some foods and beverages don't have nutritional labels. Some products have false or exaggerated advertising and claims listed on them that you shouldn't believe. Also, new research is always being done in the field of nutrition and you need to stay current or risk making less intelligent decisions on what you eat. Purchasing and reading this book is a fantastic start to your nutrition education but this new field continues to grow and there is always more to learn. Avoid learning your nutrition information from companies that are simply advertising their products or unnatural bodybuilders that have achieved their physiques through illegal drugs. Some reputable sources for you to look into include WebMD, The American Heart Association, The American College of Sports Medicine, and dozens of other academic journals.

Clip Coupons and Check Sales

You may think clipping coupons is a waste of time, but if you spend a few minutes a week on it the savings will add up! Checking out your grocery store's flyers also help to find the daily, weekly, or seasonal specials. Signing up for your vendor's email newsletter or promotions may also provide access to plenty of coupons and savings. Another great method now is signing up for your store's rewards account where they scan your card on every checkout. This will end up getting you plenty of savings throughout the store and often some additional rewards and cashback. The store gets to know what kind of products you prefer so it can stock up and you get save money. That sounds like a win-win situation to me.

Purchase Goods On Clearance

Sometimes you can get lucky and the food item that you are looking for is on clearance. This can be for several reasons like the store is overstocked, the packaging is dented, or the item is going to expire in the next month or so. As long as the quality of the item is not in question, I'd say go for it! I once bought a box of cereal that was normally $4 for $1 because the cereal box was dented. The bag on the inside was still sealed and the cereal wasn't crushed so I bought it for just a quarter of the regular price. Items like that are constantly falling off shelves, being mishandled, or dropped and this can be your ticket to extra savings. There may be a clearance isle or section in your local grocery store and you can ask the manager or a store clerk where it is.

The Water Trick

This trick works whether you are afraid of over-eating, overspending, or both. Before you go out or face the meal in question, make sure to drink about 16 oz of water beforehand so that you are filled up and your appetite is naturally decreased. You can also fill yourself up with other healthy and low calorie options such as vegetables, whole grains, a whey protein shake, coffee, tea, or other zero calorie beverage. This is an excellent tactic to use before going out to eat, out to a party, or going shopping at the grocery store. Drinking water or eating healthy food is also a much healthier and more natural alternative than taking some of the questionable and expensive appetite suppressant supplements that are out there. Not to mention drinking water is free!

Negotiate Prices

This strategy really only works with small store or restaurant owners that have the flexibility to make individual deals if they see fit. This obviously won't work at big box stores and huge chains unless you are a master negotiator. They say that everything is negotiable and food is no exception. Things that may be negotiable include items that the store is overstocked with, food that is slow to sell, freshly made breads or bagels that are a day old, or products that are getting somewhat close to their expiration date. You may be able to negotiate discounts on a large volume order or a cash deal as well. The best place to practice this is at your city or town's local food market. Learning to haggle will help not only help you save money on your food bill and it's always a good skill to have.

Get Sponsored

Do you think only professional athletes get sponsored by food companies, supplement companies, or restaurants? Think again. While you may not be able to finagle a six figure deal with Gatorade, it is definitely possible for sponsorships or partnerships to be created. If you are a member of a local sports team, look into making a deal with a local healthy restaurant. Ask them to provide healthy post-game food in exchange for free publicity or a spot on your uniforms. If you are involved with a church or charitable organization, many supermarkets or restaurants would be happy to help contribute to the cause in one way or another. One of those ways may be providing healthy and nutritious products to those running the charity and those receiving the charitable donations. It can be a win-win situation for everybody involved. There are many other deals and relationships that can create free or discounted nutrition to you and others. It may just might take a little work and persistence to get started but eventually it will pay off big time. While it may not be possible for every person or organization to get a sponsorship, you never know until you try and it never hurts to ask.

Barter

Sometimes getting food products or nutritional supplements simply requires a trade of services. I know many people that have provided their trade or expertise in exchange for the products of a store, restaurant, or supplement company owner. I've provided personal training on occasion for nutritional supplements, as long as the exchange is worthwhile to both parties. Perhaps the store, restaurant, or company owner needs the services you provide but normally couldn't afford them. They purchase or cook their products at wholesale prices and provide them to you in exchange for your product or service and everybody wins. It's not rocket science and in many situations it can be the smartest move. You may even get referrals for your quality products or services, increase your income, and then have even more money to invest in your health and fitness!

Don't Shop When You Are Hungry

This may seem like common sense but it is very important to remember. Grocery stores are systematically designed to make you buy more food than you originally planned on. They pump additional oxygen into the store and keep the lights bright to keep you alert and energetic in your shopping journey. They want you to come in for milk and eggs and leave with a shopping cart full of expensive items! If you shop when you are hungry you are almost guaranteed to purchase more food and more unhealthy foods. You might even end up buying twice as much food as you need when your rationale thought is skewed by a voracious appetite. I know I've purchased all kinds of strange and unhealthy foods in the past when I was shopping hungry. I was even aware that I was just being manipulated by the store setup and food product marketing. After I ate something I wondered why I purchased so many stupid items. Hunger is a powerful force and it will cause you to think and act irrationally.

Only Buy What You Can Carry

This is another well-known tip to make sure your grocery shopping experience doesn't get out of hand (no pun intended). When you have a big shopping cart, your natural tendency is going to be to fill it up at least somewhat. If you instead go shopping with the resolve to only purchase what you can carry with your hands or a basket, you will only purchase the bare essentials. Not only will it limit the food that you can buy, but it will give you a little more of a workout during your shopping spree! Also, by purchasing smaller amounts of food each time you will ensure that your food and meals are always fresh. It may also improve your meal planning and you will have to throw out less expired food that you forgot about. This suggestion applies more to meat, produce, and frozen items. I would not recommend this tactic if you are trying to save time and money by buying healthy food in bulk.

Spice It Up

Using herbs and spices to improve the palatability and variety of your healthy meals is very important. Eating chicken breasts, tuna, salad, pasta, veggies, etc all the time can get really old really fast and you need to change things up at least a little bit. Spices may be slightly expensive when you first purchase them but they will most likely last you a long time. They are a very affordable and convenient way to change a meal significantly with little effort. Not only are spices cheap and versatile, but they add only a negligible amount of calories and many of them have health benefits. Spices such as garlic, onion, and cinnamon all have very well documented health benefits. You can even grow your own herbs pretty cheaply and easily for more potency. Salt and pepper always work, but make sure to minimize the salt if you have high blood pressure or heart disease. Spices will help to enhance the flavor of food in the place of salt for those on a low sodium diet.

Take Advantage of Restaurant Specials

If there are specials for your favorite restaurants, take advantage of them. Lunch specials are a good way to get your favorite foods for a lower price than the dinner equivalent. You may risk being called an old geezer but you can often take advantage of the infamous Early Bird Specials for dinner at 4 or 5pm. Some days of the week offer half-priced appetizers or special meal deals which also make going out more affordable. Just make sure that the foods you are saving money on aren't also hurting your waistline. A good way to be kept in the loop on your favorite restaurant's specials and promotions is to sign up for their newsletter or email newsletter. Now you can even get notified of daily restaurant specials through Facebook and Twitter!

Go Out To Eat Less

This one is pretty much common sense but a lot of people don't use it. While you can find good bargains at restaurants like I mentioned before, odds are the more you go out to eat the more your eating expenses increase. You will definitely save significantly by eating out once or twice a week at the most and cooking the rest of your meals yourself. Also, while you can find healthy options at restaurants, chances are you will also eat less healthy the more you eat out. When you cook something yourself, you decide all the ingredients that go into it. When you go out to eat, you may not see all of the butter, sauces, sugars, and other ingredients that are added to your food to enhance the flavor. Eating out less will also make you appreciate the few times that you do go out to eat

Order Online

This tip applies mostly for purchasing nutritional supplements. Most foods aren't worth purchasing online, especially when shipping costs are factored in. In terms of nutritional supplements, there are a wide variety of vendors online that offer better prices than the local GNC or Vitamin Shoppe. There are thousands of online supplement stores out there and it is becoming an increasingly competitive industry. There are also more supplements and supplement companies coming out every year. This helps you, the consumer, because these companies must constantly have sales, specials, and price cuts to sell their inventory. Just make sure you are still getting a good bargain after you factor in the shipping costs. There are also some people that find great deals on buying healthy food in bulk online so that may be worth looking into further. Rare foods, or traditionally high-priced food items like almond butter, may be much cheaper buying straight from the manufacturer and/or in bulk than at your local store.

My Top Frugal Places For Food Shopping

- Wal-Mart
- Costco
- BJ's
- Trader Joe's
- Market Basket
- Dollar Tree
- Farmer's Markets
- CVS (supplements)
- Walgreens (supplements on clearance)
- AllStarNutrition.com (supplements)
- Bodybuilding.com (supplements)

III

Nutrition Tips

Throughout my career as a Personal Trainer I have found that for most people, eating properly is even more difficult than getting consistent and effective workouts in. Making healthy eating choices is something we all have to deal with several times a day and every day of our lives. Many people don't know what foods to eat, why to eat them, when to eat them, etc. There are also hundreds of ridiculous diets, fads, lousy nutritional supplements, myths, and just plain lies out there making it confusing for everyone. It is difficult to eat clean all the time even if you know exactly what you are doing. We need all the help we can get so use this as a guide to improve your overall nutrition. I don't expect perfect nutrition from the average person, but making a few changes and sticking with them can mean all the difference when it comes to health and physique.

It is important to educate you on the best nutritional and training methods so you will be able to workout more efficiently and with better results. Having a good physique and being healthy is largely based on your daily nutrition. You do not want to go to unhealthy extremes like under-eating or eliminating one macronutrient such as carbohydrates or fat from your diet. Fad, extreme, or yo-yo diets are not the answer. The key to nutrition is to MANIPULATE YOUR METABOLISM TO BURN MORE CALORIES! Here are some major tips to keep in mind. A few of these you may already know while others will make a major difference in your fitness level. You do not have to follow all of these guidelines all the time, which would be unrealistic. Knowing sometimes is half the battle and if you can at least follow a few of these tips it will make a significant difference!

Split Up Your Meals:

Instead of eating 2-3 big meals a day, try to go for 5-6 smaller meals throughout the day. This will prevent you from overloading you digestive system and will keep your metabolism and energy level high. This principle works in conjunction with portion control for all of your meals to avoid overeating at any one time. Try to carry around some small healthy snacks with complex carbs, protein, and fiber (nuts, health bars, fruit, veggies, granola, etc)

Good Daily Eating Example:
-Medium/large breakfast
-Light/medium snack
-Light/medium lunch
-Light snack
-Light dinner
-Very light snack before bed

Bad Daily Eating Example:
-Skip Breakfast
-Big Lunch
-Big Dinner
-Big Snack Before Bed

Eat More The First Half of The Day:

Everybody's metabolism is fastest during this time and you will burn off most of the food you eat throughout the day. A moderate-large and healthy breakfast/snack/lunch will provide you with the critical nutrients and energy you need throughout the day. Keep in mind that the "first half" of your day is relative to when you go to sleep and wake up. The first half of your day might start at 5am if you go to work early or it might start at 4pm if you work overnights. The key is to start eating right when you wake up and before you get involved with a million other tasks.

Reduce Eating At and After Dinner:

Everybody's metabolism at the end of the day slows down significantly which is why you always here things like "don't eat anything after 7pm" and so forth. That is because some of the calories you don't burn off before you go to sleep will be stored as fat overnight. This all depends of course on what foods you eat, the amount of food, what you have for dinner, when you did your workout, what type of workout you did, etc. If you are trying to lose weight then make sure to keep your after-dinner snack small. Try to make it high in protein and complex carbs, low in sugars and fats. I would recommend a bowl of oatmeal/whole grain cereal and a cup of skim milk for the average person. I encourage most people to have a small healthy snack after dinner unless they are trying to lose weight very aggressively. What you don't want to do is eat a whole bunch of junk food, sweets, or alcoholic beverages before you go to sleep.

Drink Plenty of Water:

As I mentioned earlier, this will help keep you full so you won't feel as hungry. It also helps to cleanse your system and guarantees you are more hydrated. Drink 8-16 ounces of water to naturally reduce your appetite. Also acceptable: Decaf tea, Propel, crystal light, seltzer, diet soda, etc. By having a water bottle on you all the time, you can avoid many potential dieting pitfalls. I try to keep water in my car, gym bag, gym locker, bedroom, and at my desk so I always have it on hand if necessary.

Estimating Your Caloric Requirements

When you are trying to lose or gain weight in a healthy manner, it is important to remember that there are many factors affecting bodyweight. Some of these variables include activity level, gender, age, height, weight, and obviously genetics. It is also good to keep in mind that a pound of fat is about 3,500 calories so to burn fat you must create enough of a caloric deficit through exercise and/or dieting. Utilize the Harris-Benedict Equation which uses your Basal Metabolic Rate (BMR) and incorporates an activity factor to determine your total daily energy expenditure in calories The main factor omitted by the Harris-Benedict Equation is lean body mass. Leaner bodies typically need more calories than those with a higher body fat percentage. Because of this, the Harris-Benedict Equation will be very accurate in all but the very muscular (underestimating calorie requirements) and those with very high levels of body fat (overestimating calorie requirements). The first step is to calculate your Basal Metabolic Rate (BMR):

1. Calculate Your Basal Metabolic Rate (BMR):

Standard BMR Formula

Women: BMR = 655 + (4.35 x weight in pounds) + (4.7 x height in inches) - (4.7 x age in years)
Men: BMR = 66 + (6.23 x weight in pounds) + (12.7 x height in inches) - (6.8 x age in year)

Metric BMR Formula

Women: BMR = 655 + (9.6 x weight in kilos) + (1.8 x height in cm) – (4.7 x age in years)
Men: BMR = 66 + (13.7 x weight in kilos) + (5 x height in cm) – (6.8 x age in years)

2. Apply the Harris-Benedict Principle:

To determine your total daily calorie needs, multiply your BMR by the appropriate activity factor, as follows:

Sedentary: (little or no exercise): BMR x 1.2

Lightly Active: (light exercise 1-3 days/week): BMR x 1.375

Moderately Active: (moderate exercise 3-5 days/week): BMR x 1.55

Very Active: (hard exercise/sports 6-7 days a week): BMR x 1.725

Extremely Active: (very hard exercise, double training): BMR x 1.9

(www.bmicalculator.net, 2010)

The Zig-Zag Method of Fat Loss

If you are trying to lose weight in a healthy way, this is one of the most important methods to apply to your weekly nutrition plan. The first step is calculating your estimated daily calorie requirements. Then, depending on how strict you want to diet, you reduce your calorie intake 5 or 6 days of the week. The other 1 or 2 days you eat more calories than you need. It is usually best to eat approximately 300-500 calories less than normal 5-6 days per week and the remaining 1-2 days a week you can consume 200-300 calories more than your estimated requirement. This allows you to have a "cheat" day or two when you go out to eat, etc while also keeping your metabolism from going down. If you diet everyday your metabolism will drop because your body cannot work as hard on less energy and it will conserve fat and calories. This method is much more realistic than what other extreme diets suggest and even more effective. Don't go absolutely crazy on your cheat days but try to plan them out and enjoy them knowing that they won't throw your diet off track (Hatfield, 2004).

Zig-Zag Method of Fat Loss Weekly Examples

Example #1:   **Moderate Dieting Weekly Eating Plan:**
Monday: Consume 500 Less Calories Than You Require
Tuesday: Consume 500 Less Calories Than You Require
Wednesday: Consume 500 Less Calories Than You Require
Thursday: *Consume 300 More Calories Than You Require*
(Cheat Day)
Friday: Consume 500 Less Calories Than You Require
Saturday: *Consume 300 More Calories Than You Require*
(Cheat Day)
Sunday: Consume 500 Less Calories Than You Require
Net Loss: **1,900 Calorie Deficit Per Week**

Example #2:   **Strict Dieting Weekly Eating Plan:**
Monday: Consume 500 Less Calories Than You Require
Tuesday: Consume 500 Less Calories Than You Require
Wednesday: Consume 500 Less Calories Than You Require
Thursday: Consume 500 Less Calories Than You Require
Friday: *Consume 300 More Calories Than You Require*
(Cheat Day)
Saturday: Consume 500 Less Calories Than You Require
Sunday: Consume 500 Less Calories Than You Require
Net Loss: **3,200 Calorie Deficit Per Week**

1 lb of fat − 3,500 calories

Read Nutrition Labels:

I am repeating this suggestion in this chapter for emphasis since it is that important. It is crucial to know how to read nutrition labels for improving health as well as saving money. You need to be able to figure out a serving size of the food, the main ingredients (listed in order from largest amount to least), any possible allergy concerns, and of course nutrient content. Don't let advertising convince you that a food is good. Just because a food is "diet" or "reduced fat" etc. does not mean it is healthy or any better than the original version. There are plenty of "health foods" out there that you should actually stay away from.

Sugar Only In Morning and Post-workout:

The only times it is actually beneficial to have simple quick-digesting carbohydrates is right in the morning when the body's glycogen supplies are low. At this point, and also after a workout, your metabolism is very high and the sugar will be used up right away and not stored as fat. There is nothing wrong with the occasional piece of fruit at other points in the day. If you eat too many servings of fruit or other servings of simple sugars, it may increase your bodyfat.

Consume High Fiber Foods:

High fiber foods definitely complement the "water trick" very well. Consuming foods high in fiber will help keep you satiated and less likely to overeat or eat junk. The fiber doesn't really contribute to your overall caloric intake so don't worry about that. Getting enough fiber in your diet is also important to stay regular and for overall health.

Dealing With Chocolate Cravings:

Nearly everyone loves chocolate and many of these people get cravings for it from time to time. I personally love chocolate and need to consume it in one way, shape, or form every week. My daily solution is to make a protein shake with chocolate whey or casein protein powder. As you will read in the "Frugal Supplements" chapter, I am a big fan of Dymatize's 12 Hour Elite Fudge Brownie protein powder. It tastes great, doesn't cost much, is high in quality, and will only help you in your goal to reduce bodyfat. Sometimes I also mix in some peanut butter or sugar free chocolate syrup. At worst I would buy some chocolate hard candies and suck on one or two per day when the craving strikes. You are better off consuming 50 extra calories than several hundred (or one thousand!!) with a chocolate bar, cake, etc. You could also purchase chocolate pudding which will not do any damage to your diet because it is less than 100 calories. Dark chocolate, while very high in fat and calories, can be eaten in moderation and provides some healthy antioxidants. Make sure the dark chocolate is at least 60% cacao to maximize antioxidant content and minimize added chemicals and sugar. If you absolutely have to have some chocolate junk food, consider it one of the 1-2 "cheat" days allotted per week. Just don't go overboard!

A Simple Guide to Macronutrients

What Are Macronutrients?

Macronutrients are simply the sources of calories that we can ingest. These macronutrients include carbohydrates, proteins, fats, and alcohol. A lot of people think that all calories are the same but nothing could be further from the truth. Each macronutrient is broken down and utilized by the body differently. Getting the best types of each macronutrient and the correct ratio of macronutrients will help you improve your health and fitness level greatly.

Carbohydrates:

Carbohydrates are pretty important since they are the main source of energy for your brain and muscles. A diet very low or devoid of carbohydrates may help some people lose a little weight but it will leave a person physically and mentally exhausted. A better and more realistic way is to try and consume more "good carbs" and less junk. Avoid simple sugars from foods such as soda, too much fruit juice, white bread, white rice, cookies, candy, cakes, etc. These simple sugars usually don't satisfy hunger very well so people keep large amounts of them until they are full. This can be very difficult but you should try to opt for more complex carbs when you can such as whole wheat/grain products, veggies, oatmeal, brown rice, sweet potatoes, Kashi, Total, etc. Subtract the grams of sugar from the grams of total carbohydrates to determine the amount of complex carbohydrates. Complex carbs are excellent sources of fiber as well as other important nutrients and provide long lasting energy. Each gram of carbohydrates provides 4 calories of energy. Fiber does not really provide any calories though because it is not digested significantly by the body and instead simply goes through your digestive system.

Protein:

Proteins, and their amino acid components, are the building blocks of many parts of your body including muscles. Each gram of protein provides 4 calories of energy. Adequate protein intake will help improve muscle recovery, increase metabolism, and increase satiety. Increased muscle recovery and growth will help decrease bodyfat because your muscle tissue is metabolically active and thus burns calories at all times. Foods that are good for this while being low in fat include skim milk, whey/soy/casein protein powder, eggs (especially egg whites), nuts, seeds, chicken, turkey, lean beef, fish (wild Alaskan salmon is the best!), protein bars, beef jerky, fat free cottage cheese, and fat free yogurt, etc. Protein consumed after a workout involving resistance training may also naturally increase levels of growth hormone and testosterone which can be beneficial to your bodyfat levels and physique.

Fats:

Fats should not be avoided like the plague. They are crucial for energy storage, organ protection, performance in aerobic activities, and satiety. Each gram of fat provides a massive 9 calories of energy. However, you do want to avoid saturated fats (red meat, fried foods, butter, cakes, pastries), especially trans fats which cause even more artery clogs and heart disease than regular saturated fats. Foods sold in the United States are now required to display trans fat content due to a 2006 legislation. Most companies have removed it from their foods or reduced it to such small amounts that they don't legally have to list it on their labels. In New York and many other cities they have also banned it in restaurants! Unsaturated fats, fat that comes mostly from plant sources and is liquid at room temperature, are fine for you and can actually be beneficial to heart health, cholesterol levels, and normal body maintenance. Omega-3 fatty acids are very beneficial for overall health and cholesterol levels. Good sources of fat include eggs, vegetable oils, nuts, sunflower seeds, natural peanut butter, almond butter, salmon, anchovies, mackerel, and flaxseeds.

Alcohol:

While alcohol is technically a macronutrient, it should be an extremely small percentage of your caloric intake. Each gram of alcohol provides 7 calories of energy. Unfortunately, alcohol has almost no beneficial nutrient content and has many detrimental side effects on the body. Dark beers do have some beneficial health properties but not at the expense of the alcohol and carbohydrate content in my opinion. Red wine does have some of the highly-touted antioxidant resveratrol but in my opinion it is not worth the damage from the alcohol. It is highly concentrated in resveratrol but it is not conclusive if 1 glass of red wine gives you enough for significant health improvements. You also would be consuming a lot of simple sugars with each glass of wine which is often combined with a slow metabolism late at night. One alcoholic beverage at night is not going to derail your diet. If you drink one every night or drink a larger quantity, you may be cancelling out a lot of the progress you made from other dietary or exercise improvements.

Simple vs. Complex Carbohydrates

A lot of people get confused on the subject of simple and complex carbohydrates, and as they are sometimes referred to as "Good and Bad Carbs". Using this terminology, the good carbs are the complex carbohydrates and the bad carbs are the simple carbohydrates. This is not always accurate however because sometimes simple carbohydrates are better suited for certain activities or times of day. Typically, simple carbohydrates have a higher Glycemic Index (GI) which measures its effect on your blood sugar levels compared to table sugar. This means that simple carbohydrates are more likely to spike your blood sugar levels which can lead to a subsequent crash shortly after. Complex carbohydrates take longer to digest and thus provide a more stable and longer lasting supply of blood sugar to the body. Deciding what type of carbohydrates you should be eating and when is crucial for improving your health and fitness levels. Simple carbohydrates are ideal in morning immediately after waking up as well as before, during, and after a workout. Complex carbohydrates are ideal pretty much any time except right before, during, or after a workout. Healthy examples of simple carbohydrates include fruits, 100% fruit juice, and honey. Healthy examples of complex carbohydrates include vegetables, whole grains, legumes, brown rice, and sweet potatoes.

Healthy vs. Unhealthy Fats

There is also confusion over what kinds of fats are healthy and unhealthy to consume. Originally, low-fat diets were all the rage and people would try and avoid any foods with fat in them, even if they were healthy sources. We know today that eating a diet devoid of fat will only be detrimental to your health and fitness goals. During the Atkins Diet craze, people sacrificed as many of their carbs as possible but ate as much fat as they wanted including unhealthy sources. I believe that the best goal for the average person is to find the happy medium between these two extremes. Healthy fats are usually considered to be the unsaturated fats, some of which provide Omega-3 fatty acids which can provide many healthy benefits. Unhealthy fats are usually the saturated fats, especially the trans fats which can be very damaging to your health and fitness goals. Try to keep your ratio of unsaturated : saturated fats as high as possible and avoid trans fats whenever possible. Good sources of unsaturated fats include nuts, seeds, vegetable oils, avocados, and fatty fish. Sources of saturated and trans fats include processed foods, fast food, fried food, sweets, candy, and red meat.

Complete vs. Incomplete Proteins

In my experience, people have the least understanding of the difference between complete and incomplete protein sources. A food is a complete source of proteins if it provides all of the essential amino acids for human dietary needs. Incomplete proteins provide only a fraction of the essential amino acids and therefore must be combined with other incomplete proteins to provide all the body's necessary amino acids. The problem with many vegetarian diets is that they are deficient in the amount of complete proteins since they do not consume animal products. Through smart eating and potential protein supplementation, vegetarians can definitely get enough protein and amino acids in their diet. Complete proteins are only from animal sources, soy, and quinoa. Incomplete proteins can be found in nearly all other foods and good sources include whole grains, nuts, seeds, and beans.

The Benefits of Antioxidants

Antioxidants have been getting a lot of publicity over the past decade or so. They have often been touted as miraculous natural solutions to prevent aging and various diseases. But what exactly are antioxidants and just how effective are they? Antioxidants are molecules that prevent free radicals, or oxidizing agents, from causing cellular damage. These free radicals are thought to be what causes aging and various medical conditions including cancer. Free radicals come from pollution, stress, chemicals, and other sources. While natural and common in human biology, excessive free radical exposure may cause accelerated aging or disease. By ingesting or topically applying antioxidants, the damage done by free radicals may be minimized and overall health may be improved. Some of the most common antioxidants include Vitamin A, Beta Cartone, Vitamin C, Vitamin E, Zinc, Selenium, resveratrol (found in grapes and red wine), ECGC, glutathione, Lutein, and lycopene and more.

There are new experiments coming out all the time on the promise and disappointments of antioxidants for health. While there are thousands of more experiments to be done to confirm the benefits and shortcomings of various antioxidants, there is plenty of promise so far. Many alternative and trial treatments for cancer, AIDS, and other major chemical conditions have utilized various antioxidants with some success. These foods and supplements may not be miracle drugs but for many people they can be safe and useful ways to improve overall health. I would encourage you to cover your bases and consume a wide variety of antioxidants by eating large amounts of colorful fruits, vegetables, teas, and spices. Purchasing, ingesting, and topically applying very large amounts of antioxidants however may not be beneficial to your health and may even be detrimental. Vitamins A and E can potentially accumulate in your system to toxic levels and nutritional supplements and herbs may not be pure or as described on the label. I usually only recommend Vitamin C supplements (since it is water soluble) and tea/tea extract supplements for extra antioxidants.

Performance Nutrition Basics For Youths & Teens

1) **Always Eat Breakfast!**
   This will provide the fuel you need for the day, important for maintaining high energy levels in school, on field/court, and gym class. If you skip breakfast, you'll end up dragging most of the day.

2) **Drink Lots of Water Throughout the Day!**
   Always have a bottle of water with you to stay hydrated and healthy.

3) **Eat enough protein!**
   Important for muscle growth/repair after exercise

4) **Eat your fruits and vegetables!**
   Provides a good source of water, fiber, as well as vital vitamins and minerals.

5) **Eat healthy snacks throughout the day!**
   Helps keep your energy levels up and your muscles fueled, eat many smaller meals throughout the day and not just 2-3 large meals.

6) **Avoid Fast Food and Junk Food!**
   These are unhealthy choices & add body fat

7) **During a workout, drink water or Gatorade!**
   Stay hydrated, no sodas before, during, or after practice!!!

8) **After a workout, replenish Protein and Carbs!**
   Ex) Skim Milk, Chocolate Milk, Carnation Instant Breakfast, Gatorade, and/or fruit)

9) **Bring Your Own Lunch**
   Some schools are offering much healthier breakfast and lunch alternatives to purchase but most offerings aren't very healthy. Try to bring your own healthy meals to school and avoid that Salisbury Steak.

10) **Eat Healthier Desserts**
    Try to make the switch to low fat ice-cream, fruit, and yogurt.

Performance Nutrition For Teens/Adults

The following outline is what I would recommend for the average teenager (that has already hit puberty) or adult. Manipulating your carbohydrate and protein consumption before, during, and after a workout can help to maximize the performance and recovery of your workout, competition, race, etc. Your carbohydrates are your main source of energy and you need to time them correctly depending on your physical activity and goals. Complex carbohydrates need to be consumed hours before your workout because they take much longer to digest and have a higher fiber content (Conley et al, 1996). Several hours before your workout you may want to consume some healthy fat as well if you are going to engage in a long endurance workout because you may require more energy from fat sources. Bodybuilders and individuals looking to lose weight usually do not need to worry about consuming healthy fats before a workout. Simple carbohydrates may be taken within an hour before your workout for a quick-digesting source of energy. Easily digested protein such as whey protein powder may be ingested before a workout if you are trying to maintain or gain lean muscle mass (Almada et al, 2007). During a workout, I recommend drinking water unless you are sweating profusely, working out for a prolonged period of time, working out in the heat, or seriously trying to put on weight. In this case, I would recommend drinking a diluted sports drink like Gatorade. When I say diluted, I would drink only 1/3 or ½ Gatorade and the rest would be water. Some bodybuilders like to drink caffeine, carbohydrate drinks, or protein shakes during their workout but I think this is overkill and a waste of money. Within 15 minutes after your workout is complete, you need to replenish the carbohydrates you burned for energy and create a more anabolic (muscle-building) environment for your muscles. A quick digesting protein such as whey protein powder immediately post-workout may help to enhance muscle recovery and promote muscle growth and increases in natural anabolic hormone levels (Campbell et al, 2007).

For An Athlete/Runner:

3 Hours Pre-Workout:	Large serving of complex carbohydrates, some healthy fat and protein
1 Hour Pre-Workout:	Serving of simple carbohydrates
During Workout:	Diluted sports drink or water
Post-Workout:	About 50-60 grams of simple carbs and 20 grams of whey protein

For A Bodybuilder:

3 Hours Pre-Workout:	Serving of complex carbohydrates, protein shake
1 Hour Pre-Workout:	Protein shake and/or creatine product, caffeine
During Workout:	Water
Post-Workout:	0-60 grams of simple carbs and 35 grams of whey protein

For Someone Trying To Lose Weight:

3 Hours Pre-Workout:	Serving of complex carbohydrates, lean protein
1 Hour Pre-Workout:	Whey protein powder in water, caffeine
During Workout:	Water
Post-Workout:	Whey protein powder in water

Performance Nutrition For Endurance Athletes

Pre-Race Nutrition:

2 Weeks Out-	-1.5 Weeks of low-carbohydrate eating, higher fat and protein -This allows for glycogen depletion and fat loading (major source of energy in endurance events) while maintaining calories/muscle mass
3 Days Out-	-All 3 days eat very large amounts of carbohydrates, especially complex carbs -This allows for carbohydrate loading to maximize glycogen stores for the race -Consume moderate protein and fat during these days
3-4 Hours Pre-Race-	-High Carbohydrate meal low in fat and protein (oatmeal and fruit)
1 Hour Pre-Race-	-Piece of Fruit
15 Min Pre-Race-	-Water, Gatorade or Goo (optional)
During Race-	-Water/Gatorade every few miles -Goo Packet every 8 miles running
Post-Race-	-Rehydrate thoroughly, consume some simple carbohydrates in the form of fruit and/or Gatorade. Consume 20-30 grams of whey protein powder in water.
After Race Day-	-Plenty of carbohydrates to replenish glycogen stores, protein for muscle recovery, and Omega-3 fatty acids for anti-inflammatory benefits. High calories.

Healthy Lifestyle Tips

Get 8 Hours Of Sleep A Night

There is a lot of debate and conflicting study results when it comes to how much sleep people need for minimum and optimum performance. Different people are going to require different amounts of sleep but my opinion is you shouldn't skimp on it. Adequate sleep will help you recover fully from your workouts and other stresses in your life. Getting insufficient sleep can throw off your hormonal balance leading to stress, lower energy levels, muscle loss, and weight gain. Poor sleep habits can prevent you from making significant improvements in your health and fitness levels and can lead to other health issues. If you can't seem to make time for a good night's sleep, you may need to reevaluate your commitments and priorities. Luckily, proper eating and exercise habits may improve your ability to get to sleep as well as the quality of your sleep.

Eliminate Unnecessary Stress

Stress is a killer. Increased stress leads to weight gain, increased blood pressure, muscle atrophy (breakdown), and overall poor eating habits. It can also lead to poor sleeping habits or be brought on by those poor sleeping habits. The stress hormone cortisol plays a negative role on your metabolism and recovery when sleep habits are poor and there is chronic high stress. Try to stay organized, find some time to relax, and even try controlled breathing and meditating. Get rid of the negative influences in your life that are causing frustration and holding you back from your potential. There are many frugal ways to try and reduce stress. Try out a few yoga, meditation, or tai chi classes.

There are thousands of cheap yoga and stress-relieving dvds out there and even free videos. You may also want to check your health insurance to see if it covers chiropractice, massage therapy, or accupuncture treatments.

Make Health and Fitness a Major Priority

This one is the key to success when trying to achieve your health and fitness goals. Try to stick with your program and think of the dozens of reasons why it is beneficial to you. Make a list of all the reasons to live healthy if you need to. This is where the Goals List in the beginning of the book comes in. Any time you feel like you are losing motivation or discipline, revisit the list of your goals and the reasons you want and need to improve your health and fitness. If you need to, make photocopies of your Goals List and plaster them up places that you will constantly see them such as your desk, your car dashboard, your bathroom, or your fridge. This will help to remind you and may subconsciously help you make healthier decisions. If you do not make fitness a major priority in your life and you can't cnjoy it, you will not be able to keep it up. That is setting yourself up for failure.

No Smoking

This is an obvious no-no. Smoking will reduce your cardiovascular strength and endurance, reduce your energy levels, and lower your immune system. Your body will spend its resources trying to clean out the toxins inhaled and have less energy and nutrients to spare for muscle maintenance and exercise recovery. If you smoke you will most likely have less motivation to workout and even less energy to workout if you do make it to the gym. Even your recovery will be stunted or delayed. If you have an addiction to cigarettes, you need to do everything in your power to cut back and break the habit or your health and fitness levels will be held back considerably. Talk to your doctor about medication options, Smoking also costs an incredible amount of money these days and the taxes just keep going up and up! That's not frugal or smart for anyone trying to make an improvement in their quality of life.

How To Avoid Derailing Your Diet

Stock Up On Healthy Snacks:
One of the most important ways to ensure that you are
eating healthy foods is to always have them around you.
That means keep healthy food and snacks on hand in your
house, at your desk, at work, in your car, in your gym
locker, in your briefcase, or wherever you need them. If you
have good healthy food available, you will be less likely to
waste money and ruin your diet on fast food, vending
machines, snack bars, and other similar options.

Don't Keep Junk Food On Hand:
It's hard to eat junk food when you don't have any to eat in
the first place! Sure you can leave your home or office to go
purchase some, but you are less likely to sabotage your diet
if it isn't around staring you in the face. This means that you
need to take any junk food in your home, office, car, bag,
purse, etc and get rid of it. When I say get rid of it, I mean
throw it away or give it away and not eat it all. From now
on, don't purchase any more junk food ever again. Don't
accept cakes, cookies, and other treats from friends or
family as a gift. Just thank them and politely refuse. If they
insist, find another home for it or throw it away. Get rid of
the temptation and the cravings will subside eventually. This
works better for some people than others but I guarantee it
will help out at least a little bit.

Don't Stress Out About Imperfection:
Everybody is going to hit a snag in their dieting at one point
or another. The key is to remain calm and not beat yourself
up over it. Some people will get so guilty or stressed out
about eating a little bit of junk food that they'll either dwell
on it too long or just call off the whole diet. Don't use a less
than perfect meal as an excuse to get upset or give up. The
right thing to do is write it off as a cheat meal or cheat day
and get back on the right track the next meal. You can

always make up for it by eating a little less or working out a little longer the next day. The Frugal Diet is about improving in the grand scheme of things and one meal or day won't make or break that. It's not about eating perfectly all the time and you need to cut yourself a little slack if you mess up. Be patient and remember dieting isn't a sprint, it's a marathon.

Recognize Your Weaknesses and Plan Accordingly:
We all have weaknesses when it comes to certain foods, drinks, situations, or locations. For example, I know that I will most likely eat any food in my home so I plan accordingly by only having healthy foods at home. Everybody's dieting weaknesses are different and first you need to determine what they are. Do you tend to eat too much when you go out to eat or when you are with friends? Do you tend to drink too much when you go to parties or in certain situations? Do you eat when you are stressed out or depressed? There are many different scenarios that are unique to each person. You can either prepare as much as possible for all of these scenarios or you can try to simply avoid them as much as possible. That all depends on your lifestyle and commitment but you need to figure out a game plan before these events occur to prevent or minimize a major setback.

Treat Yourself To At Least 1 Cheat Meal A Week:
You need to unwind and enjoy your favorite food or beverage at least once in awhile or you might go crazy. That one cheat meal or cheat day that is built in to The Frugal Diet will help keep you sane while still allowing you to make overall health and fitness improvements. Feel free to make it a special occasion and plan it out to maximize your enjoyment. Go to your favorite restaurant and enjoy!

Nutrition Myths Busted

Myth #1: Carbs Are The Enemy!

Truth: Carbohydrates are extremely important for everyone no matter what their fitness goals may be. As the primary source of fuel for your brain and muscles, a person cannot function on a carb-free diet without adverse mental and physical effects, especially if they are physically active. The trick is to stick to complex carbohydrates that do not cause the spike in blood sugar and are less likely to promote fat storage. These slower digesting carbs will provide more stable energy throughout the day and you will not "crash" after about an hour like you may if you chugged a bottle of soda. Complex carbs will also offer many more nutrients such as fiber, vitamins, and minerals that the processed simple sugars are lacking. If you are trying to lose weight, you may want to reduce your overall carbohydrate intake a little bit but not at the expense of your day to day functioning.

Myth #2: Fat Is Bad For You!

Truth: Again, like carbohydrates, fat is essential for normal function and performance and it is simply a matter of getting the right type of fat in your diet. A lower-fat diet may help you lose some weight but don't try to completely eliminate fat from your diet (which is pretty much impossible anyways). Stick to the unsaturated fats and those high in Omega-3 fatty acids. This usually means reducing the amount of fried, processed, and junk foods you consume. Saturated fats are usually solid at room temperature and unsaturated fats are usually liquid at room temperature.

Myth #3: Diet, Reduced Fat, and Sugar-Free Foods Are Good For You

Truth: Just because a food says that it is "Low Fat", "Diet", etc. does not necessarily mean that it is good for you. "Low Fat", "Reduced Fat", and "Fat Free" products may compensate with extra sugar. Conversely, "Low Carb" and "Sugar Free" products may compensate with higher amounts of fat. This may be done to preserve the taste or consistency of the product. Sodium may also be added to these products to maintain taste. I'm not saying all of these products aren't better than their originals, I'm just saying that the only way to know for sure is to check the labels and know what to look for. I use many diet, fat free, and sugar free products daily but I have also seen a lot of inferior diet products out there that should be avoided. Most food companies have websites with nutrition information for their products so you can compare and contrast for yourself online or just at the grocery store.

Myth #4: Skipping Breakfast Will Help Me Lose Weight

Truth: Skipping breakfast will not help you lose weight and it isn't a healthy idea. Skipping the most important meal of the day can even make you gain bodyfat in the long run! By skipping breakfast, your body has no source of fuel and your metabolism will slow down accordingly so your body will burn less calories. Your body may even start breaking down some of its muscle tissue for energy which will also lower your metabolism. You will also feel sluggish and tired throughout the day. Most people will make up for a skipped breakfast with unhealthy snacks or a massive lunch. The feeling of decreased energy from a skipped breakfast will also take away from your motivation to hit the gym later. Also, coffee is not breakfast!

Myth #5: Meat Is Terrible For You

Truth: Meat has been getting a bad reputation for decades from doctors and vegetarians but it can be a very healthy part of a balanced diet if eaten correctly. It is true that fatty cuts of red meat tend to raise bodyfat and cholesterol levels, but lean cuts of pork and beef contain excellent amounts of protein and other nutrients. The type and amount of meat ultimately determine how healthy it will be for your diet. Unless you are morally opposed, I don't see anything wrong with having plenty of chicken and turkey or a few servings of lean red meat per week. I say everything in moderation.

The New Food Pyramid

The original food pyramid from 1992 has been redesigned and updated several times recently due to new nutritional studies. I think the new food pyramids are also a response to all the dieting crazes, and increased obesity trends that have been so prevalent over the last couple decades. It is now more specific on the serving sizes of certain food groups such as proteins. It encourages lactose free products and/or calcium supplements for those that are lactose intolerant. Fish, poultry, beans, and eggs are highlighted as the lean proteins and nuts/legumes provide protein and heart healthy fats/fiber. It clarifies that you should focus on consuming whole grain foods instead of just breads and cereals in general. It also finally makes the distinction that fruits are good but fruit juice is usually not and should be used sparingly. There are many versions of the food pyramid for different age groups and populations but the official one is now known as "MyPyramid" and can found on www.mypyramid.gov.

Frequently Asked Nutrition Questions

What Are The Differences Between Foods and Supplements?

There are many differences between food items and dietary supplements. The main difference is that food is inspected and regulated by the FDA and dietary supplements are not. Dietary supplements often make claims on their products but none of the statements are approved by the FDA. Even the ingredients and purity are not overseen by the FDA so the potential for contaminated or exaggerated content is much higher with dietary supplements. You are probably taking larger risks by consuming dietary supplements but keep in mind the FDA doesn't exactly have a perfect track record either.

What Are Sugar Alcohols?

Sugar alcohols are used as sweeteners because they pass through your digestive system relatively intact, therefore not contributing any calories to your body. For this reason they are considered similar to sugar-free sweeteners because they do not have a significant effect on your caloric intake or blood sugar levels. Sugar alcohols are often used as sweeteners in foods and chewing gum, especially in Europe. Sugar alcohols have been known to cause stomach and digestive discomfort in some people, especially when consumed in large amounts. I also see a lot of sugar alcohols in protein bars that want to limit the amount of "impact carbs" (total carbs minus fiber and sugar alcohol content) while giving their bar a sweeter flavor. My opinion on sugar alcohols is to avoid consuming too much at once. One or two pieces of gum are fine but some products have way too many sugar alcohols for your body to handle at once. They certainly aren't healthy but then again no artificial sweetener is beneficial to your health.

Why Are Some Nutrients and Information Listed On Some Food and Supplement Labels And Not Others?

The FDA only requires some of the basic nutrients to be included on food labels so some labels have only the minimum requirements. This is often due to limited space on the food label. A prime example of this is peanut butter. Many companies just put a couple of micronutrients on the label and do not include all of the B-Vitamins, Vitamin E, or mineral content found in peanuts. If you weren't an expert on foods, how would you know that it contained these nutrients? Not every company, product, or consumer cares about how much Vitamin E or Riboflavin there is in a product, or the ratio of polyunsaturated fats to monounsaturated fats. There are sometimes new policies and legislation that changes what food labels are required to include. For example, all food products now are required to list their trans fat content if they contain over a certain amount per serving. Since the general public is more a little more educated on nutrition, there seems to be more nutrition information listed on food labels now than there used to be including specific fiber types, micronutrients, herbal ingredients, caffeine content, and mention of specific ingredients that many individuals have allergies or intolerance. Because of the success of portion control and points programs/diets such as Weight Watchers, many foods also list it's equivalent value of a starch, protein, or fat source. I personally like to see as much nutritional information on a food product as possible to know what I am putting into my body.

What Is The Difference Between Soluble & Insoluble Fiber?

Both of these types of dietary fiber are important for you to consume in your daily diet. Getting at least your daily value of fiber can help you avoid a whole laundry list of health problems. Soluble fiber is fermented in the digestive system by bacteria while insoluble fiber simply goes through your system absorbing water and softening your stool. There are countless other subtle differences and benefits of both types of fiber but you should mainly focus on getting in plenty of both types for overall health. Most Americans aren't getting nearly enough fiber in their diet so most of us should be concerned with simply getting more quantity. Eating healthy foods such as whole grains, nuts, seeds, beans, fruits, and vegetables will give you plenty of both types of fiber for optimal health.

What Is The Difference Between Monounsaturated and Polyunsaturated Fat?

Both polyunsaturated and monounsaturated fats are considered "heart healthy" or beneficial fats compared to their saturated and trans fat counterparts. Polyunsaturated fats have more than one double bond in the fatty acid chain while monounsaturated fats have only one double bond in the fatty acid chain. Monounsaturated fatty acids are found in foods such as olive oil, canola oil, teaseed oil, nuts, and avocadoes. Polyunsaturated fats are found in foods such as fish, algae, krill, leafy greens, nuts, seeds, and cheese. There are various studies out that suggest varying effects on cancer metastasis and insulin resistance, among other things, but the studies are by no means conclusive. (Vessby et al, 2001). My opinion is not to worry about the subtle differences between these unsaturated fats, just try to consume more of these and less of the saturated and trans fats to cover your bases.

How Do Low Carb Diets Work?

Low carb diets can work for some people but they must be done correctly and over a long period of time. Be reducing your carbohydrate intake, your body is basically forced to burn more bodyfat instead of glycogen. The only problem is, carbohydrates are the main source of energy for the brain and your muscles. That means, on top of the cravings, you will also have to deal with very low energy levels and decreased physical or mental performance. While low carbohydrate diets can help you lose some fat, it isn't smart or healthy to have your brain and muscles essentially running on fumes. I do not recommend very low carb diets to most people unless they are competitive bodybuilders or fitness models that must lose as much bodyfat as possible.

Can You Ever Take In Too Much Protein?

Contrary to what you hear from some bodybuilders, yes you can ingest too much protein. Everybody can handle different amounts of protein because of varying age, gender, muscle mass, activity level, activity type, and genetics. If you ingest more than your body can process at once, it can be stored as bodyfat and detrimental to kidney health. Always make sure you are hydrated when taking protein supplements or consuming larger amounts of protein-containing food. Bodybuilders on anabolic steroids and/or human growth hormone can process higher amounts of protein than a normal person so that is one reason why their diets are so high in protein and you shouldn't replicate them. While everybody is different, my opinion is to limit protein intake to no more than 30 grams per hour and no more than 1 gram per pound of bodyweight per day. There are dozens, if not hundreds of numbers, ratios, and equations for optimal protein consumption out there but that is just my personal opinion. In terms of being conservative or liberal on protein consumption, I would put myself as slightly liberal on the scale. You need extra calories no matter what in order to gain muscle mass, but contrary to many scientific studies out there I believe you also need at least a little extra protein consumption as well.

Do Energy Drinks Really Work?

Energy drinks give you temporary energy from caffeine and sugar (unless it is a sugar-free energy drink like I prefer). The caffeine increases your metabolism and thus gives you more energy and mental alertness. It may give you energy during certain activities but not always during high intensity exercise, especially if it dehydrates you. The massive amount of sugar content in regular energy drinks can spike your blood sugar and give you an initial rush of energy, but then you will crash around an hour later. The sugar-free energy drinks rely solely on the caffeine and other stimulant content to provide you with extra energy, even though you will also crash after the caffeine high ends. Energy drinks may give you a temporary energy boost but they are not very healthy and no match for a healthy diet (including complex carbs) and workout program.

Do "Fat Burners" Really Work?

This is another yes and no answer. Fat burners are usually just glorified and expensive caffeine supplements that raise your metabolism through a stimulant effect. Caffeine increases your heart rate, fat burning, and energy levels so in the long run this can contribute to extra pounds of fat being lost. Fat burning supplements, such as Stacker 2 or Hydroxycut, also contain smaller amounts of other ingredients such as Green Tea Extract, Chromium, Taurine, amino acids, and other herbal ingredients and micronutrients to supposedly increase the fat burning potential of the supplement. While these ingredients may help you burn fat to an extent, I don't think they are worth the massive increase in price from just regular caffeine, coffee, etc. They can also cause headaches, stomach aches, jitters, heart palpitations, and potentially heart attacks or strokes in some people. It really depends on your health, medical conditions, weight, age, and caffeine tolerance but these should be taken with caution or simply avoided.

What is Normal, Healthy Weight Loss?

Healthy weight loss for the average person is about 1-2 lbs of fat loss per week. Any more than that is usually due to loss of water weight and sometimes a partial loss of muscle mass. If you lose water weight, you will be dehydrated and you will end up putting this weight right back on as soon as you drink anything. If you lose muscle mass, your metabolism will go down and you will end up burning less fat in the long run. The 1-2 lbs of fat loss per week is a generalization though so it will vary depending on your age, gender, genetics, metabolism, activity level, diet, etc. If you have a lot of weight to lose, you may easily lose more than 1-2 lbs of fat per week. If you start out in excellent shape, it may take a month or more of proper diet and exercise to lose 1-2 lbs of fat.

How Do I Get Rid of my Belly and Hip Fat?

Unfortunately there is no such thing as "spot-treating" when it comes to working out problem areas. That means, doing a thousand crunches a day won't get you a six pack and doing a thousand leg raises a day won't get you tight hips. The same goes for dieting. You can't eat certain foods or calorie amounts to directly reduce your waistline or hips. The natural fat deposit areas for men is usually in the stomach and for women in the hips so that means most people will have more fat to lose from those places. You may lose the same amount of fat from your midsection as you are from your arms, legs, shoulders, etc but it might not be as noticeable since those other areas had less fat to begin with. Only an effective and customized nutrition and exercise regimen will allow you to reduce the bodyfat from these problem areas for the long term. It takes time so don't get impatient if your desired bodyparts don't get smaller or leaner immediately. You probably didn't put on all that bodyfat overnight so it won't come off overnight either.

How To Read a Food Label

As I mentioned several times earlier in this book, educating yourself on nutrition and learning how to read a food label may be the most important skill of all for improving health and fitness. Nearly all foods and supplements are required to post their ingredients and nutrition content so you can make the right choices. Some of the most important information is to interpret the ingredient list, serving sizes, calories, calories from fat, amount of fat, amount of carbohydrates, amount of protein, sodium content, cholesterol content, and the micronutrient (vitamin and mineral) content. To help make this easier to understand, I will give you several examples of common foods and how to analyze the nutritional content. For each food I will give you a quick breakdown on the major factors and an overall risk-benefit analysis to determine if it is a worthwhile food choice.

Example #1: A Good Carbohydrate Source

Nutrition Facts

Serving Size (290g)
Servings Per Container

Amount Per Serving

Calories 200   Calories from Fat 35

% Daily Value*

Total Fat 3.5g	**5%**
Saturated Fat 0.5g	**3%**
Trans Fat 0g	
Cholesterol 0mg	**0%**
Sodium 5mg	**0%**
Total Carbohydrate 36g	**12%**
Dietary Fiber 5g	**20%**
Sugars 1g	
Protein 7g	

Vitamin A 0%	•	Vitamin C 0%
Calcium 4%	•	Iron 15%

*Percent Daily Values are based on a 2,000 calorie diet. Your daily values may be higher or lower depending on your calorie needs.

		Calories	2,000	2,500
Total Fat	Less Than		65g	80g
Saturated Fat	Less Than		20g	25g
Cholesterol	Less Than		300mg	300 mg
Sodium	Less Than		2,400mg	2,400mg
Total Carbohydrate			300g	375g
Dietary Fiber			25g	30g

Calories per gram:
  Fat 9 • Carbohydrate 4 • Protein 4

This food label is for oatmeal and you can tell pretty quickly that it is an excellent source of carbohydrates. Out of the total of 36 grams of carbohydrates, only 1 gram is sugar! Also note the 5 grams of fiber which is a very large amount for one serving. Another excellent thing to note is the 7 grams of protein, a pretty good amount for a carbohydrate source. There is also no sodium, cholesterol, or saturated fat (.5 grams is negligible). The ingredients list is not included on this label but it only contains 100% rolled oats so there are no artificial flavors, additives, preservatives, or filler. If you compare this information to the nutrition content of processed and sweetened oatmeal, you will find it is vastly superior in every way.

Example #2: A Poor Carbohydrate Source

Nutrition Facts

Serving Size: 3/4 cup (27g)

Amount Per Serving

Calories 108   Calories from Fat 9

	% Daily Value*
Total Fat 1.05 g	**2%**
Saturated Fat 0.24 g	**1%**
Trans Fat	
Cholesterol 0 mg	**0%**
Sodium 157.68 mg	**7%**
Potassium 29.7 mg	**1%**
Total Carbohydrate 23.73 g	**8%**
Dietary Fiber 0.19 g	**1%**
Sugars 11.88 g	
Sugar Alcohols	
Protein 0.97 g	
Vitamin A 750.06 IU	15%
Vitamin C 0 mg	0%
Calcium 1.35 mg	0%
Iron 1.8 mg	10%

This is the nutrition label for Post Fruity Pebbles and you can easily note the lack of nutritional content. Out of the 23.73 grams of total carbohydrates, about half of them are sugar and there is almost no fiber or protein! This is because nearly all of the nutrients have been processed out of it to make the cereal sweet, light, crispy, and have a longer shelf life. There is also a decent amount of added sodium for flavor and no other redeeming nutrients. This would never be a good choice of carbohydrates unless you were starving to death so avoid the many similar cereals out there as best you can. Opt for a much more nutrient dense cereal such as Kashi or Total for a better source of carbohydrates.

Example #3: A Good Fat Choice

Nutrition Facts

Serving Size 2 Tbsp (32g)

Amount Per Serving

Calories 200 Calories from Fat 150

	% Daily Value*
Total Fat 16g	25%
Saturated Fat 2g	10%
Trans Fat 0g	0%
Cholesterol 0mg	0%
Sodium 120mg	5%
Total Carbohydrate 7g	2%
Dietary Fiber 2g	9%
Sugars 2g	
Protein 7g	

Vitamin A 0%	Vitamin C 0%
Calcium 0%	Iron 0%

*Percent Daily Values are based on a 2,000 calorie diet. Your daily values may be higher or lower depending on your calorie needs:

	Calories:	2,000	2,500
Total Fat	Less than	65g	80g
Saturated Fat	Less than	20g	25g
Trans Fat			
Cholesterol	Less than	300mg	300mg
Sodium	Less than	2,400 mg	2,400mg
Potassium		3,500mg	3,500mg
Total Carbohydrate		300g	375g
Dietary Fiber		25g	30g

INGREDIENTS: PEANUTS, SALT

This is the nutritional label for a jar of natural peanut butter. The most obvious way you can tell it is an excellent fat source is the ratio of saturated fat to total fat. The ratio is 1:8 so only 12.5% of the fat content is saturated, the rest is pretty much heart healthy. Also note that the only two ingredients in this natural peanut butter are peanuts and salt. Regular peanut butter from the big name brands usually contains partially-hydrogenated oils (a source of trans fats), added sugar, and several other added ingredients for consistency, taste, and shelf life. You can also see that this provides a decent amount of protein and some fiber as well.

Example #4: A Poor Fat Choice

Nutrition Facts

Serving Size: 3 blocks (37g)

Amount Per Serving	
Calories 189	Calories from Fat 88

	% Daily Value*
Total Fat 9.83 g	**15%**
Saturated Fat 5.89 g	**29%**
Trans Fat	
Cholesterol 4.07 mg	**1%**
Sodium 72.52 mg	**3%**
Potassium 120.25 mg	**3%**
Total Carbohydrate 23.67 g	**8%**
Dietary Fiber 0.81 g	**3%**
Sugars 19.44 g	
Sugar Alcohols	
Protein 2.45 g	
Vitamin A 37.74 IU	1%
Vitamin C 0.3 mg	1%
Calcium 58.46 mg	6%
Iron 0.39 mg	2%

This is the nutritional content for a Hershey's Krackel bar which is obviously not too good for you. Over half of the fat content is saturated fat and a serving of this bar also provides tons of empty sugar. There is no significant redeeming protein, fiber, or nutrients in the bar as well. Another big variable to note is that the serving size is "3 blocks" so depending on the size of the bar, there may be many serving sizes. If the bar consists of 9 blocks and you eat a whole block, multiply all the fat, sugar, and calories by 3 to get your total intake!

Example #5: A Good Protein Source

Nutrition Facts	Amount/Serving	% DV*	Amount/Serving	% DV*
Serv. Size 1/4 can (55g) **Servings** 4	Total Fat 2g	3%	Total Carb. 0g	0%
	Sat. Fat 0g	0%	Dietary Fiber 0g	
Calories 60 Fat Cal. 20	Cholest. 15mg	6%	Sugars 0g	
* Percent Daily Values (DV) are based on a 2,000 calorie diet.	Sodium 30mg	1%	Protein 14g	
	Vit.A 0% • Vit.C 0% • Calcium 0% • Iron 4%			

This is the nutritional label for a typical can of tuna which can be a frugal and healthy dietary staple. About 2/3 of the calorie content in this tuna is from protein and because it is from an animal source, you know it is complete protein. Because there is so little fat and no carbohydrates, the overall calorie content is very low which is great for dieting. There is no sugar and no saturated fat. The fat content in the tuna provides a decent amount of omega-3 fatty acids. There are no carbohydrates so it will mesh with even a low-carb diet. There is a little cholesterol but otherwise this can of tuna is an ideal source of protein.

Example #6: A Poor Protein Source

Macaroni and Cheese

Nutrition Facts

Serving Size 1 cup (228g)
Servings Per Container 2

Amount Per Serving

Calories 250	Calories from Fat 110

	% Daily Value*
Total Fat 12g	**18%**
Saturated Fat 3g	**15%**
Cholesterol 30mg	**10%**
Sodium 470mg	**20%**
Total Carbohydrate 31g	**10%**
Dietary Fiber 0g	**0%**
Sugars 5g	
Protein 5g	

Vitamin A	**4%**
Vitamin C	**2%**
Calcium	**20%**
Iron	**4%**

* Percent Daily Values are based on a 2,000 calorie diet.
Your Daily Values may be higher or lower depending on
your calorie needs.

		Calories	2,000	2,500
Total Fat	Less than	65g	80g
Sat Fat	Less than	20g	25g
Cholesterol	Less than	300mg	300mg
Sodium	Less than	2,400mg	2,400mg
Total Carbohydrate		300g	375g
Dietary Fiber		25g	30g

This is the nutritional label for a macaroni and cheese
product and as you can see it has more negatives than
positives. First off, this 250 calorie serving provides only 5
grams of protein. Since about half of this protein is from the
noodles and not the cheese, that means half of this measly
amount of protein is incomplete as well. It provides a very
large amount of fat (25% of the fat being saturated), no
fiber, and tons of cholesterol and sodium. Cheese can be a
good source of protein but the minimal and fake amount of
cheese and added filler make this a no-no if you are looking
for a high quality source of protein.

Potential Cholesterol-Lowering Foods

The more of these you get in (except excessive alcohol), the better it may be for your HDL, LDL, and Total Serum Cholesterol. The HDL (or high density lipoproteins) are the good cholesterol, the LDL (or low density lipoproteins) are the bad cholesterol, and they both add up to your total serum cholesterol. You want your total serum cholesterol significantly below 200. Also, the higher the ratio of HDL to LDL, the better your cholesterol is. While more studies are needed to confirm the benefits of the following foods on cholesterol levels, there are plenty of personal testimonies and hypothesis to encourage consumption. Try to incorporate at least a few of these foods everyday! (and avoid sodium!)

-Avocadoes
-Almonds
-Blueberries
-Alcohol/Red Wine (1 Drink)
-Lentils
-Beans
-Oats
-Salmon
-Flaxseed
-Garlic

Mike's Thoughts On Artificial Sweeteners

There are many different sweeteners out there now and it is difficult to decide which ones, if any, are appropriate for you and your goals. The old sweeteners of Sweet and Low and Equal now have the more expensive option of Splenda to compete with. There are also a wide variety of other "healthier" sweetener options such as agave nectar, stevia, xylitol, and others which are significantly more expensive and less researched (Szalavltz, 2006). The reason all of these artificial sweeteners were created in the first place was to create zero calorie alternatives to table sugar, high fructose corn syrup, etc. There are many conflicting studies and opinions out there about artificial sweeteners causing health problems including cancer (Karstadt 2006). Many other problems such as headaches, migraines, and digestive problems have also been associated with various artificial sweeteners (Journal of Head and Face Pain, 2007). While ideally it is best to avoid artificial sweeteners and sources high in table sugar/high fructose corn syrup, that is not always realistic for everyone and sometimes you have to choose the lesser of two evils. In my opinion, I would rather consume artificial sweeteners in my food or beverage instead of 40 grams of traditional sugar or high fructose corn syrup that your body can't process. Large amounts of high fructose corn syrup is not natural and any type of sugar will cause a large spike in your blood sugar levels. This blood sugar spike can cause more proven health problems such as increased risk of obesity, increased cravings for other junk food, and negative effects on insulin levels and sensitivity. My advice is to try and eat as much natural food so you can minimize sweeteners of all types. None of them are good for your health but you can make up your own decision on which sweetener choice makes sense to you. More research is being conducted on these sweeteners to determine the short term and long term effects. Unfortunately, artificial sweeteners are a multi-billion dollar industry so sometimes the studies and results may be sponsored or skewed by companies with a vested interest. I think only time will tell just how dangerous or negligible these artificial sweeteners are and how they compare to regular sugar or high fructose corn syrup.

What (Not) To Eat At Restaurants

The Frugal Diet is primarily about purchasing and cooking snacks and meals from the supermarket. You can minimize going out to eat significantly with proper cooking, storage, preparation, and planning. That being said, everybody goes out to eat or travels at least occasionally so you need to know what to prepare for. Usually going out to eat will translate into setback in your health and fitness regimen. Going out to eat is a fun and special treat, not normally a time or place where you are fully concerned with the nutritional value of your order. Chances are you will be with friends and family, distracted from what you are eating, and potentially drinking alcoholic beverages. You are surrounded with delicious foods and smells and you will most likely order and eat more than you should. There is nothing wrong with having a good time and enjoying the foods you love but don't try and kid yourself that eating one type of burger at McDonalds will help you lose weight compared to another burger choice. I personally just order pretty much whatever I feel like at restaurants and try to eat healthy and clean the rest of the week. Although there are a few exceptions, try to avoid fast food restaurants except as a last resort.

I was originally going to do an "Eat This, Not This" section of foods that are and aren't acceptable at common restaurants. The problem is there is just so little in the former category that I would personally endorse consuming. Almost every food or drink served at a restaurant is either unhealthy, expensive, or both. Instead, I want to keep things simple and generalized. Stick with the basic foods and meals that are included in this book, or offerings that are similar. When in doubt, you can't really go wrong with a light salad, grilled chicken, grilled salmon, vegetables, water, tea, tuna, stir fry, tofu, whole grains, whole wheat options, and fruit. Perhaps in a later edition of this book I will compile a list of acceptable healthy and frugal foods when you are eating out but currently the list is miniscule.

Mike's Short List of
Healthier Frugal Restaurant Foods

- **Unlimited Soup and Salad**
  (Olive Garden)

- **Low Fat Turkey Bacon Breakfast Sandwich**
  (Starbucks)

- **Grilled Chicken Sandwich w/ lettuce and tomato**
  (McDonalds)

- **Chicken Noodle Soup and Whole Grain Baguette**
  (Panera)

- **Grilled Chicken Bucket**
  (Kentucky Fried Chicken)

- **Stir-Fries with Vegetables, Salmon or Chicken, and Brown Rice**
  (Fresh City)

- **Grilled Chicken Sandwiches with Vegetables on Whole Wheat Bread**
  (Subway)

V

Top 25 Frugal Powerfoods

I'm sure I didn't come up with the term "powerfoods" but nonetheless here are some foods that I think are extremely effective, healthy, and versatile foods for almost everyone out there, regardless of your goals. I take into account price for most of these choices since these foods should be purchased consistently. Everybody is different but I think the average person would make major improvements in their health and physique if they ate more of the following foods. Now without further ado, my favorite powerfoods (in no particular order).

1. Oatmeal
If I had to pick just one frugal food, oatmeal would probably be it. Now I'm not talking about the oatmeal that is refined and comes with all the sugar and maple syrup

already in it that they market to little kids. When I say oatmeal I mean 100% rolled oats. One of the cheapest foods on the list, 100% rolled oats are an incredible source of complex carbohydrates. You can purchase several pounds of oatmeal for just a few dollars and your carbohydrates are covered for weeks. With no sugars and no saturated fats, there is no downside to this food choice. Oatmeal contains plenty of fiber (soluble and insoluble) for overall digestive health along with several grams of protein as well. If you have a severe wheat allergy or intolerance (celiac disease) oatmeal may not be right for you because often the oats may be contaminated with wheat from the manufacturing process.

2. Tuna

Tuna is an excellent and cheap source of complete protein without any significant fat or carbohydrates. It comes in a convenient can which takes care of almost half of your protein requirements for the day. Tuna also has some other nutrients including Omega-3 Fatty Acids and selenium. The only problem is that over the decades tuna has become more and more corrupted by mercury. This means that there may be small amounts of mercury in most cans of tuna so it should be eaten only in moderation. I would recommend still eating tuna but limit your intake to 2-3 cans per week. Tuna is much cheaper than salmon and nearly as healthy except it contains less Omega-3 Fatty Acids. Salmon is the nutritionally superior choice but the price of tuna is right.

3. Eggs/Egg Whites

Another bodybuilding staple, eggs and egg whites are both fantastic for high-quality sources of protein. I wouldn't recommend chugging 8 raw eggs Rocky-style (can you say Salmonella?) but I encourage nearly everyone to get eggs or egg whites in their diet. Egg whites are nearly pure protein and are excellent for those looking to stay extra lean and can be prepared very easily from liquid form in Egg-Beaters. I recommend eggs over egg whites for clients unless they are really having trouble losing weight because of the more complete nutrition they provide. Eggs with yokes provide excellent sources of B-vitamins, Omega-3 Fatty Acids, and Lutein for eye health. The Omega-3 Fatty Acids in egg yokes also helps to makes up for their high cholesterol contents. You can purchase eggs from cage-free and grass fed chickens for a slightly higher price and they have a higher ratio of omega-3 fatty acids to total fat content.

4. Whole Grain Cereals

Whole grain cereals, such as Kashi and Total, provide excellent sources of slow-digesting complex carbohydrates. The whole grains also provide excellent sources of fiber and micronutrients without much or any fat, cholesterol, or processed sugar. You can purchase store-brand or generic whole grain cereal for very low prices and each box will provide you with a large amount of servings. There are plenty of other smaller brand name cereals in the organic food section but they are often $5 or more for a small box and aren't usually worth the extra cost. Many whole grain cereals are also fortified with extra vitamins and minerals for even more versatility. My personal favorite is Kashi Heart to Heart Honey Toasted cereal because it has plenty of nutritional value and minimal sugar. You can also snack on it right from the box. If you add in fruit, milk, and nuts you will have a complete and healthy meal.

5. Whole Grain Breads

Whole grain breads are another staple for a healthy and frugal diet. A loaf of generic whole grain bread will only cost you about $2 but it will provide you with at least half a dozen servings of complex carbohydrates, fiber, and micronutrients. I like to keep things fresh by varying between whole wheat bread, multigrain bread, whole grain bread, whole wheat English muffins, and whole grain bagels. Whole grain pita bread also makes a great affordable snack with hummus or for wraps. Make sure to check the nutritional label though to see just how many whole grains are in it. Be wary of wheat or multigrain breads that contain unwanted ingredients such as high fructose corn syrup. It's so easy to just grab a whole grain bread product and spread on some natural peanut butter or whatever you prefer for a cheap and healthy snack on the go. Often times I get lazy and just eat whole grain toast with natural peanut butter or pita bread and hummus as my meals or snack.

6. Peanuts/ Natural Peanut Butter

Peanuts and peanut butter are excellent sources of healthy fats, fiber, protein, vitamins, and minerals. They are both extremely cheap options and very easy to eat as a snack or with other healthy foods. Although the cost is slightly more expensive, I would opt for natural peanut butter instead of the traditional Skippy or Jiffy product. These more traditional peanut butter products have hydrogenated oils, a source of trans fats, for consistency and added sugars for enhanced flavor. Natural peanut butter just has peanuts and salt and is a much cleaner food nutritionally. If you purchase peanuts, make sure that there are no other added ingredients except for peanuts and salt. You can obviously purchase peanuts or peanut butter without added salt if you have high blood pressure or heart disease. I eat scoops of natural peanut butter plain and right out of the jar if I get hungry. While almonds have a slight nutritional and allergy advantage over peanuts, they also cost more than twice as much so peanuts and peanut butter are the frugal winners.

7. Skim Milk

Believe those commercials about milk doing a body good! Low fat or skim is a very cheap, high quality complete source of slow-digesting proteins. Skim milk also contains high amounts of potassium, calcium, and Vitamin D making it a very versatile beverage. It does contain 13 grams of lactose (milk sugars) per serving but these sugars do not spike blood sugar and insulin levels as much as those found in sweets, fruit juice, and soda. A gallon of skim milk is $3 or less at most supermarkets and provides 8 servings. I've been drinking tons of skim milk for my whole life and I give it credit for a significant amount of my muscle growth and repair. Make sure that you purchase milk that says on the label that it is from cows that are steroid, growth hormone, and antibiotic free. There are also more expensive brand name fat free milk that have higher amounts of protein light-blocking containers. These are good choices to try out but you need to determine whether they are worth the extra cost. Also make sure to check and compare the expiration dates to the other gallons of milk to get the freshest possible option.

8. Chicken Breasts

A perennial weight loss and bodybuilding staple, chicken breasts are nearly fat free and an excellent source of protein. Because "chicken tastes like everything" it can be cooked in a variety of ways with various other foods and spices so it does not get so boring day after day. Purchase chicken breasts in large quantities, cook them in large quantities, and you have high quality protein for the whole week! Before you grill them up, cut off any significant pieces of fatty tissue to make them even leaner choices. Try to purchase frozen chicken breasts as opposed to already cooked and sliced options as those will be much more expensive. Check the label to make sure that they are at least 97% lean and are not treated with growth hormones, steroids, and antibiotics.

9. Whole Grain Pasta

Whole grain pasta is a very versatile and inexpensive excellent source of complex carbohydrates and long-lasting energy. A box of generic whole grain pasta costs about $2 and provides several servings of nutrient density. There are also plenty of variations, shapes, and types to keep you from getting bored. Pasta is so easy to cook that there is no excuse for not getting enough whole grains for lunch or dinner. Whole grain pastas are especially important for endurance athletes looking to maximize their stores of muscle glycogen for optimal performance. If you are aggressively trying to lose weight, limit your pasta consumption at or after dinner to one serving at the very most.

10. Coffee

Coffee is good for you?! Yes it is actually. The reason that coffee gets such a bad reputation is because so many people add massive amounts of cream and sugar to it or accompany it with unhealthy companions such as donuts or cigarettes. The rich and expensive mochachinos and custom drinks can also total over 500 calories which can be kryptonite for your diet. Also, drinking more than 2 or 3 cups a day is not necessarily good for you and will boost your caffeine tolerance considerably. Coffee by itself, or accompanied with skim milk and a zero calorie sweetener, can help to increase your metabolism and fat-burning. Coffee is also a natural appetite suppressant so it can help reduce your cravings for junk food. It even provides a small amount of naturally occurring antioxidants! Coffee can be a very cheap source of caffeine if you purchase and make it yourself, or simply order a regular coffee at your local café. It will burn a hole in your pocket though if you go to the local Starbucks every day though and order designer drinks. Coffee should be avoided or consumed in moderation if you have hypertension, heart disease, or caffeine sensitivity. Avoid drinking caffeinated coffee beyond the afternoon to avoid disrupted sleeping habits.

11. Tea

Tea doesn't contain any calories and it can be very useful for supplementing most weight-loss programs. Green tea is the most touted tea for health benefits out there but you can purchase about 100 generic black tea or orange pekoe tea bags for $1 at any grocery store. That's hard to beat! All teas provide significant amounts of antioxidants so you can't really go wrong in my opinion. Green tea is versatile because it has the powerful antioxidant ECGC that may boost your immune system and metabolism. Tea also contains small-moderate amounts of caffeine per cup which can improve utilization of fat for energy and improve overall metabolism. Caffeinated tea usually has about 1/3 of the caffeine content of the leading premium coffee. One or two cups a day will add up over the weeks, especially 30-60 minutes before doing cardio. Limit, avoid, or switch to decaffeinated tea in the evening so sleeping habits are not disturbed.

12. Vegetable Oils

Vegetable oils such as canola and olive oil provide an excellent supply of unsaturated fats. They are excellent for cooking and are a much healthier alternative to butter or other animal-derived fats. Vegetable oils are extremely cheap to purchase, especially in large containers, and allow you to make your own salad dressings. Margarine and butter alternatives are a high percentage of vegetable oils and therefore have less saturated fats and more Omega-3 fatty acids. Pure vegetable oil is better for you than the butter alternatives but I love them so making the switch from real butter is a big upgrade. Most of the margarine products now have changed their ingredients to eliminate partially hydrogenated oils that are sources of trans fats. There are also affordable brand names that offer light margarine products with even less calories. You can purchase 3-4 pound tubs of margarine products for $5 or less and they will last you for quite a long time. There are numerous studies out praising the benefits of vegetable oils and they are a staple on the new food pyramids. Eating plans such as The Mediterranean Diet tout the wonders of vegetable oils as one of the major reasons why inhabitants of that region have such low blood pressure, cholesterol, and incidence of heart disease.

13. Tomatoes

Good old tomatoes are an excellent source of the powerful antioxidant lycopene which is also important in men for prostate health. Tomatoes have some simple sugar content but the fiber, water, and antioxidant content is enough to get it on this list. I would encourage most people, especially men over 40 who are at risk for prostate abnormalities, to consume tomatoes almost everyday. Tomatoes that are locally grown seem to look and taste much better than those imported. Fresh tomatoes are the best but tomato sauce or tomato juice can be beneficial as well.

14. Flaxseeds and Wheat Germ

These are grouped together due to their similar health benefits, cost, and many uses. Flaxseeds are excellent sources of heart healthy Omega-3 Fatty Acids as well as fiber. Flaxseeds have no sugar and negligible saturated fats and can be easily added in whole or ground form to oatmeal, salads, protein shakes, breads, or spreads. They have little actual flavor so you can usually add them or mix them to anything for an extra nutritional boost. Wheat germ is a delicious, crunchy, and nutrient-packed topping you can add to plenty of salads, sandwiches, protein shakes, and other meals. It is packed with healthy fats, fiber, protein, and micronutrients. A large container is very inexpensive and will last you a long time.

15. Spinach and Kale

There is a reason that Popeye always ate his spinach! In reality, it isn't much of a muscle builder but it is a very affordable source of powerful antioxidants and fiber. While it won't make you strong and muscular directly, increasing your antioxidants and overall health can certainly help give you better gains in the gym or on the field. Kale is a very similar leafy green and provides very high concentrations of nutrients. Spinach and Kale are vastly superior to the iceberg lettuce that is found in so many salads. Add in spinach to your salads and sandwiches to kick the nutrition up a notch for pennies a serving.

16. Yogurt and Cottage Cheese

I've grouped these two together because they are both cheap, delicious, and convenient sources of complete protein, calcium, and vitamin D. Yogurt can also be a great source of live healthy bacteria cultures that can improve digestive health. It's a cheap, convenient, and delicious snack whether you are on the go, at the office, or even to enjoy slowly with nuts, fruit, or flaxseed toppings. Cottage cheese can be purchased in large containers pretty cheaply, there are plenty of competing brands, and there are low-fat or fat free options. Buy in bulk for extra savings or buy small containers to eat high quality protein on the go. With these two excellent options, you might want to bring a cooler with you on the go or invest in that mini fridge for your office.

17. Purple Grapes

Grapes are excellent and affordable sources of fiber, water, anthocyanins, flavenoids, and the powerful antioxidant resveratrol. Green grapes are not a source of resveratrol so I would try to eat more purple grapes than green. This is the same reason why red wine is touted as such a health tonic and white wine isn't. Trust me when I recommend that you get your resveratrol from purple grapes, and raisins if necessary, and not from copious amounts of red wine. The former has plenty of other nutrients and health benefits while the latter's high alcohol content will pretty much cancel out any real benefits gained. Also, I'd recommend sticking with purple grapes and raisins and avoiding the resveratrol and grapeseed extract dietary supplements until more studies are done to determine if they are worthwhile or not. If necessary, bring a box or two of raisins with you on the go for a light and healthy snack.

18. Chick Peas and Hummus

Chick peas, the main ingredient in hummus, are very cheap to purchase by the can and provide excellent sources of healthy fats, fiber, and protein for your diet. You can also add chick peas to salads to make them more filling and flavorful. One of the best things about chick peas is that you can just eat or prepare them right out of the container, no preparation required! Convenient, delicious, and nutritious indeed. Hummus, a product of mostly chickpeas, is slightly more expensive to purchase but even more convenient for eating with vegetables and whole grain breads or crackers. You can also make your own hummus very cheaply and easily, there are recipes for homemade hummus later in this book.

19. Carrots

Carrots are very cheap, low in calories, and packed with important nutrients. Carrots have a very high concentration of beta carotene, an antioxidant that is crucial for eye health. They also include high fiber content and many other micronutrients for overall health. Add them to all kinds of soups and salads, steam them, or just munch on them raw. Sorry but carrot cake doesn't count!

20. Sweet Potatoes

Sweet potatoes are an excellent form of slow-digesting, complex carbohydrates. Sweet potatoes do not spike your blood sugar like their more common counterpart and are an excellent carbohydrate source for anyone trying to lose bodyfat. They also include many other micronutrients and even antioxidants. They are very cheap to buy and an easy addition to any lunch or dinner. If you are aggressively trying to lose, limit yourself to one sweet potato at or after dinner at the most due to its high (but healthy) carbohydrate content.

21. Brown Rice

Brown rice provides a very cheap source of complex carbohydrates and fiber that is a versatile addition to many meals. It must be cooked a little longer than more traditional white rice but making the switch is a huge upgrade. Brown rice will not cause the large spike in blood sugar that its white counterpart will and instead provides a long steady blood sugar level. Brown rice is only slightly more expensive and harder to find than white rice but the extra pennies you pay will pay off huge healthy dividends. Some people complain that they don't like the flavor or texture as much as white rice but I promise you will get used to it. More and more people and restaurants are finally starting to break tradition to make the switch to brown rice for health reasons.

22. Soybeans

This plant source of complete proteins is good first thing in the morning or post-workout because it is quickly broken down and absorbed by the body. Soy also has healthy fats, no cholesterol, and provides heart healthy flavenoids that reduce cholesterol levels. Soybeans are very versatile and quite affordable complete proteins that everyone can enjoy regardless of meat-eating status. Common forms of soy include edamame and tofu. Soy milk is also a high-quality nutritional product but it is significantly more expensive than skim milk so it is not included in the Top 25 foods and products. There is a myth that consuming soy products will raise estrogen levels in men but that has been proven to be false. Soy protein in any form is safe and healthy to consume for men and women alike.

23. Broccoli

Broccoli provides excellent sources of fiber, water, and powerful antioxidants. The more broccoli and other green cruciferous vegetables, that you consume, the better shape your immune and digestive systems will be in and the easier it will be to lose weight. The fiber content in broccoli helps to fill you up with minimal calories. Broccoli goes great with pasta, chicken, and many other healthy frugal meals so it should be easy to get in several servings per week. Try to add it to your dinners or snack on them with hummus throughout the day.

24. Blueberries

Blueberries have long been touted as having large amounts of powerful antioxidants. They are also excellent sources of water and fiber. In my opinion, blueberries are best eaten with breakfast or post-workout so that the simple carbohydrates are immediately utilized by the body. They go great blended up in protein smoothies. There is also nothing wrong with having some as a snack in between meals as long as you don't eat a whole container at once. Sometimes they are not the cheapest fruit out there, especially when they aren't in season, but they are usually affordable enough to consume on a consistent basis along with other fruits.

25. Watermelon

This makes the list for the same reasons as tomatoes. Watermelon has some simple sugars as does any fruit but that is outweighed greatly by its water, fiber, and antioxidant content. It has such a high percentage of water content that the calorie content is very small. Watermelon has plenty of Lycopene content just like tomatoes and is a lot more refreshing on a hot summer day. You can buy a half or whole watermelon pretty cheaply which will provide plenty of servings for you and your guests.

Frugal Food Runner-Ups

1. Most Other Fruits

Many of our everyday fruits such as apples, oranges, pears, apricots, strawberries, raspberries, mangoes, cherries, bananas, grapefruits, etc are very cheap and excellent dietary staples. While each fruit has its own specific health benefits and cost, consuming 2-3 servings per day of fresh fruit in general will help to significantly improve your overall health. Just make sure you don't have too many pieces of fruit late in the day, at once, or before you go to sleep due to their high carbohydrate content.

2. Celery

Celery is another excellent frugal dietary staple. It is an excellent source of water, fiber, and has very low calorie content. It is famous for requiring more calories to chew and digest than it actually contains. Not everyone knows this but celery may also be a powerful vasodilator (blood vessel relaxer) that may lower blood pressure. Celery is almost never a bad decision to add to a meal or have as a snack. Try it by itself, with hummus, or natural peanut butter.

3. Beans

Beans are a cheap and often overlooked nutritional staple for anyone no matter what their fitness goals may be. Dry beans are considered by most to be the healthiest, some of the best being kidney beans, lima beans, pinto beans, and navy beans. They are very nutritionally dense foods packed with complex carbohydrates, fiber, protein, B-Vitamins, and minerals. They also antioxidants and fill you up so you are less likely to eat junk food. Obviously you want to avoid them in the form of refried beans or in fatty burritos.

4. Quinoa

Quinoa is a seed that is a very healthy and cheap food choice. It is also gluten-free so it is an excellent source of complex carbohydrates for those with Celiac. This staple food, often confused as a grain, has all of the essential amino acids making it a rare plant source of complete protein. That makes it an essential staple next to soy for any vegetarian. Quinoa also contains plenty of fiber and minerals for overall health.

5. Water

Water is probably the most important frugal food choice of all since our bodies are about 2/3 water. I didn't want to include it in the Top 25 however since it doesn't contain any calories and also sounds kind of lame. Water is crucial for health, performance, and weight loss no matter how you look at it. Drink as much as you can each day, especially since it is free!

Fantastic Foods That Didn't Make The Frugal Cut

1. Salmon

A little bit more expensive than most other items on the list, but Salmon provides an excellent source of complete proteins as well as a significant amount of Omega-3 Fatty Acids. Salmon is a phenomenal food, the only very minor shortcomings include its moderate cholesterol content and that a large amount of salmon on the market come from fish farms. Choose Wild Alaskan Salmon if possible for the best nutritional value. Unfortunately, the highest quality of salmon is also usually the more expensive kind. If you find salmon for an excellent price, it is most likely the farmed salmon so make sure to double check the food label or the advertisement. Occasionally there are sales on salmon making it more affordable I have included a few salmon recipes later on in this book.

2. Shrimp

Shrimp is an excellent source of almost pure protein. There is very low fat content, the only real downside is that it is very high in cholesterol. Shrimp gets a bad reputation sometimes because it is often accompanied with plates of pasta, rich creamy sauces, or plenty of tartar sauce. Buying shrimp when it is on sale or for special occasions is a good snack or meal that is high in protein and tastes great. At weddings and other formal events, I make sure to head right to the shrimp platter and stock up. Sometimes shrimp will go on sale, and some people eat small amounts of shrimp unlike myself, so I have included a few shrimp recipes later on in this book.

3. Acai Berries

While I think acai berries have recently been touted a little too much as super-antioxidants, they are still excellent foods to add to your diet. While they might not cure all diseases and help you lose 20 lbs, they are worth buying if you have the extra money to spend. Acai berries aren't sold in a lot of stores and the acai berry nutritional supplements are at least moderately expensive. There are countless acai berry supplements weight loss drinks but it is not conclusive whether these products give you the same benefits as the acai berries themselves. You are better off purchasing grapes, blueberries, or green tea instead of acai berries to get in your antioxidants if you are on a budget.

4. Almonds/Almond Butter

Almonds are probably the best nut to snack on because of a very low percentage of saturated fat content and a lower carbohydrate content than most other nuts. Almonds are also very high in Vitamin E and other micronutrients. Almond butter is usually very expensive but it has a delicious sweet and toasty taste. Almonds are great as a snack or to add some healthy fat to a meal which is important to improve satiety and fat-soluble vitamin absorption. If almonds or almond butter are too expensive, natural peanut butter or plain peanuts are a good substitute. If you buy them in bulk and eat them slowly, a bag of almonds will last you a long time and provide you with several high quality snacks.

5. Soy Milk

Unless you are lactose intolerant or vegan, I would recommend drinking skim milk instead because it is about 1/3 of the cost. That being said, soy milk is still very good for you and not outrageously priced. Soy is one of the only major plant sources of complete proteins which makes it crucial for vegetarians. It is good first thing in the morning or post-workout because it is quickly broken down and absorbed by the body. Soy also has healthy fats, no cholesterol, and provides heart healthy flavenoids that reduce cholesterol levels. Soymilk can be purchased in several delicious flavors with added sugar or in plain form with less sugar than milk. If you don't drink regular milk, I'd highly recommend adding soy milk to your diet. Don't bother purchasing rice or almond milk since neither of them provide any significant protein.

VI

Frugalicious Recipes

<u>Cooking Tips:</u>

-Substitute soy milk or Lactaid for skim milk if lactose intolerant.
-1% or 2% milk may be used if weight loss isn't primary goal
-Use a salt substitute or spices if you have high blood pressure,
cholesterol, or heart disease
-Use non-dairy vegetable oil spreads to substitute for butter or
margarine if lactose intolerant.
-Read labels on ingredients for any allergy alerts
-Nutritional content will vary based on the ingredients/amounts
- Raw eggs may contain salmonella and should be avoided.
-Cook with iron or non-toxic pans for a healthier results.
-Fully cook eggs and beef to prevent E. coli or salmonella.
-Wash all produce thoroughly before eating and cooking
-Degrees measured in Fahrenheit unless otherwise noted
-Have fun, try something new, and get creative with these recipes

<u>Breakfast Recipes</u>

Eggs-cellent Scrambled Eggs
By Michael J. Schiemer

Ingredients:
Non-Stick Vegetable Oil Spray
4 Eggs (Egg Whites if trying to lose weight)
1tsp Garlic Powder
½ Cup Kraft Fat-Free Shredded Cheddar Cheese
¼ Cup Skim Milk (optional)

Instructions:
Crack 4 eggs or however many you desire and beat them in a bowel with a fork or whisk. You can also add in the quarter cup of skim milk if you'd like and mix it in thoroughly. Heat up a frying pan on the stove to medium. Spray pan thoroughly with non-stick vegetable oil spray. Sprinkle garlic powder into the pan and then immediately add the eggs before the garlic powder burns. Scramble the eggs, put them on your plate, and top with however much low fat or fat free shredded cheese. Enjoy this very high protein, almost carb-free snack/meal.

Broccoli Cheddar Omelette
By Michael J. Schiemer

Ingredients:
Non-Stick Vegetable Oil Spray
3 Eggs (Egg Whites if trying to lose weight)
2/3 Cup Broccoli
2/3 Cup Kraft Fat-Free Shredded Cheddar Cheese
2/3 Cup Kraft Fat-Free Shredded Mozarella Cheese

Instructions:
Crack 3 eggs and beat them in a bowl with a fork or whisk. Heat up a frying pan on the stove to medium. Have your cup of broccoli and cups of cheese ready. Spray pan thoroughly with non-stick vegetable oil spray. Pour beaten eggs into frying pan, cover the whole surface of the pan, and allow the eggs to solidify at least halfway before adding broccoli and cheeses to the middle. After eggs have solidified, fold the egg over the broccoli and cheeses then press down to ensure it is closed. Cook for another 30 seconds and then flip over and press down with the spatula. Repeat if needed and cook until desired texture.

Lean and Mean Breakfast Sandwich
By Michael J. Schiemer

Ingredients:
Whole Grain English Muffin
Non-Stick Vegetable Oil Spray
1-2 Eggs (Egg Whites if trying to lose weight)
1-2 Strips Turkey Bacon
1tsp Garlic Powder
Fat Free Cheese (Shredded or 1-2 slices)
¼ Cup Skim Milk (optional)

Instructions:
Scramble eggs or egg whites as shown above (garlic powder and skim milk optional) while you toast your whole grain English muffins. You can use the same pan as the scrambled eggs to grill up the turkey bacon or you can microwave it if you have to (doesn't taste as good though). Put the eggs, turkey bacon, and some fat free cheese on the English muffin and eat as a delicious and nutritious sandwich.

Mike's Protein Pancakes
By Michael J. Schiemer

Makes: 12 pancakes

Ingredients:
1 1/2 cups oatmeal
1 1/2 cups whole wheat flour
2 tsp baking soda
1 tsp baking powder
1/2 tsp salt
1 1/2 cups buttermilk
1 cup skim milk
1/4 cup vegetable oil
1 egg
1/3 cup sugar or Splenda
3 TBSP chopped walnuts or pecans (optional)
2 TBSP ground flaxseeds (optional)

Instructions:
Grind the oats in a blender or food processor until fine. In a large bowl, combine the ground oats, whole wheat flour, baking soda, baking powder, and salt. In another bowl, combine buttermilk, milk, oil, egg, and sugar/Splenda with an electric mixer until smooth. Mix wet ingredients into the dry. Stir in chopped nuts and/or flaxseeds if desired. Lightly oil a skillet or griddle and preheat it to medium heat. Ladle 1/3 cup of the batter onto the hot skillet. Cook the pancakes for 2 to 4 minutes per side, or until brown. Store additional pancakes for later and reheat if necessary. Eat with margarine, cinnamon, fruit, and/or sugar free maple syrup.

Manic Double Blueberry Pancakes
By Crissy Kreuger

Ingredients:
2 cups whole wheat pastry flour
1 tsp baking soda
2.5 cups buttermilk or low-fat milk
2 Eggs
4 tsp Butter or Vegetable Oil Butter Spread
2 pints of blueberries

Instructions:
In a large bowl mix two cups of the flour and 1 tsp of baking soda. Add 2.5 cups of the buttermilk or low fat milk. Then add 2 eggs and mix well. Use a nonstick green pan if possible and you only need to coat pan for the first pancake to avoid frying. Add the blueberries to batter and cook. Top off with fresh fruit, butter/margarine, and maple syrup.

Egg Sandwich
By Chef Corin Szostek

Ingredients:
3 eggs
Vegetable Oil Non-Stick Spray
2 Pieces whole grain bread, bagel, or English Muffins
Onions
Low Fat Cheese

Instructions:
First spray your fry pan with non-stick cooking spray and then crack the eggs over the pan and let cook. Stir frequently so they don't burn and stick. Start on high and reduce to medium or low and cook to desired amount of time. Top with onions and low fat cheese.

Guiltless Blueberry Banana Protein Muffins
By Chef Corin Szostek

Makes: 12 Muffins

Ingredients:
1.5 cups oat bran
6 egg whites
.5 cup canned pumpkin
.5 cups all natural unsweetened applesauce
1 tsp cinnamon
cap full of vanilla extract
1 scoop protein powder (preferably Vanilla)
1 cup granular Splenda
1 banana mashed
1.5 cups fresh or frozen blueberries

Instructions:
Preheat oven to 375 degrees, and prepare a muffin tin by spraying it with non-stick vegetable oil spray. Use paper muffin paper cups/liners. Combine applesauce, egg whites, pumpkin, banana and vanilla extract in a bowl and mix well with blender. Combine the dry ingredients in a separate bowl gently (don't crush the blueberries). Once both mixtures are thoroughly combined, add the dry ingredients to the wet gradually. Once incorporated, pour batter into the prepared muffin tin. Bake for 17-20 minutes at 375 degrees (or until toothpick comes out clean).

Approximate Nutritional Values: Calories: 80 Fat: 1.5 g, Carbs: 15 g, Protein: 7 g

Oat Bran Muffins
By Chef Corin Szostek

Ingredients:
2 1/2 cups Oat Bran (uncooked)
1/4 cup raisins
2 teaspoons baking powder
1/2 teaspoon salt (optional)
2 egg whites or whole eggs
3/4 fat free skim milk
1/2 cup honey or maple syrup (sugar free if desired)
2 tablespoons extra virgin olive oil

Instructions:
Heat oven to 425 degrees F. Coat 12 medium muffin cups (get the paper muffin baking liner cups) with vegetable oil cooking spray. Combine all dry ingredients, mix well. Blend liquids together, stirring slowly. Add dry ingredients and stir until dry ingredients are moistened. Fill prepared muffin cups until almost full. Bake for approximately 10 to 12 minutes until golden brown and serve.

Ezekial French Toast
By Chef Corin Szostek

Ingredients:
2 Slices Ezekial Bread
¼ Cup liquid Egg Whites
1 tsp Vanilla Extract
Dash of Cinnamon
1 tsp Agave Nectar
Sugar Free Maple Syrup

Instructions:
Pour egg whites into a bowl and add vanilla extract, cinnamon, and agave nectar. Coat the Ezekial Bread with the egg white mixture and then fry in a pan until crispy or as desired. Top with sugar free maple syrup and/or fruit.

Classic Whole Wheat Protein Pancake
By Chef Corin Szostek

Ingredients:
2 eggs, well beaten
1   1/4 c. milk
3/4 c. whole wheat flour
2 t. baking powder
1/2 t. salt (optional)
1/2 t. Splenda
1 scoop protein powder
1 tbsp ground flaxseed
1-2 scoops of natural peanut butter
Fruit (optional)

Instructions:
Beat together eggs, milk and oil. Mix together flour, baking powder, salt and sugar. Stir into egg mixture until all ingredients are well blended. Cook on hot greased griddle or pan on stove (spray pan with cooking spray). Serve with your choice of toppings.

Blueberry Muffins
By Chef Corin Szostek

Ingredients:

2 cups whole wheat flour
1/2 teaspoon salt (optional)
1/2 teaspoon cinnamon
1 Egg
3 tablespoons baking soda
1/4 cup sugar or Splenda
1 cup fresh or frozen blueberries
1 cup skim milk
1/2 jar of blueberry preserve (sugar free if you desire)

Instructions:

Mix flour with dry ingredients in a bowl. Stir in blueberries. In a separate bowl beat eggs, milk, and oil. Add to it the flour mixture and stir just to blend. Fill 3 inch muffin tins that are greased or lined with paper baking cups, 2/3 full. Bake at 400 degrees Fahrenheit for 20 to 25 minutes. When muffins are done put 1/2 teaspoon of blueberry preserves on top in center of muffin.

Applesauce Muffins
By Chef Corin Szostek

Ingredients:
2 cups whole wheat flour
1/2 c. sugar or Splenda
2 t. baking powder
1/2 t. baking soda
1/4 tsp cinnamon
1/2 c. unsweetened natural applesauce
1 egg
1/2 c skim milk
1/3 cup extra virgin olive oil
1/2 t. salt (optional)

Instructions:
Preheat oven to 375 degrees Fahrenheit. In a mixing bowl combine flour, sugar, salt and cinnamon. Make a well in the center. Combine remaining ingredients all at once, mixing only until dry ingredients are moistened. Spoon into greased muffin tins, filling 2/3 full. Bake 15-20 min or until golden brown.

Banana Bread
By Chef Corin Szostek

Ingredients:

2 eggs

1/3 cups shortening or extra virgin olive oil

2 ripe bananas

2/3 cups sugar or Splenda

1 3/4 cups sifted whole wheat flour

3/4 teaspoon baking soda

1 1/4 teaspoons cream of tartar

1/2 teaspoon salt (optional)

Instructions:

Start over at moderate (350 degree f.) Grease 8-4 inch loaf pan. Combine eggs, shortening, bananas and sugar in glass container or blender. Cover and blend about 30 seconds or until smooth. Sift dry ingredients together into mixing bowl. Pour blender combination over dry ingredients. Stir thoroughly until combined. Pour into greased loaf pan. Bake about 45 minutes or until lightly browned. Turn out of pan to scoop onto cake rack.

High Protein Oatmeal
By Chef Corin Szostek

Ingredients:

Quick Oats

Oat Bran

Whole Grain Cereal of your choice

Natural Peanut Butter

Sugar Free Maple Syrup or Honey, Splenda (optional)

Fruit of your choice

Instructions:

Mix the oatmeal, oat bran, and whole grain cereal with water, add a scoop of peanut butter, then toppings. Microwave for 55 seconds. Stir thoroughly, add fruit.

Lunch & Dinner Recipes

My Favorite Chili
By Chef Mark Brambilla

Ingredients:
1/2 cup red wine
2 T. cumin
16 oz black beans
2 large jalapeno chili, minced
1/3 cup chili powder
28 oz whole tomatoes
2 oz pork butt
1 lb beef stew meat
3 garlic cloves, minced
2 green bell peppers
2 white onions
3 T. olive oil

Instructions:
Sauté veggies, remove, and sauté meat for 10 minutes until no longer pink. Return veggies, tomatoes with liquid, spices, jalapenos, and simmer covered for about 1 hour when meat falls apart. Add black beans and red wine. Simmer until chili thickens about 30 minutes. Serve with cheese, fat free sour cream, onions, etc.

Soft Chicken Tacos
By Joanne Koch

Makes: 4

Ingredients:
¾ lb skinless/boneless chicken breasts
1 tsp ground cumin
1 can 8 oz stewed tomatoes
¼ cup salsa
1 scallion thinly sliced
8 flour whole wheat tortilla (7 inch) warmed in oven
1 cup shredded lettuce
1 tomato chopped
4 oz light shredded cheese for tacos (1 cup)
¼ cup chopped cilantro

Instructions:
This recipe prep time is about 10 minutes and the cooking time is about 20 minutes. In large skillet over medium heat, arrange chicken in one layer. Season with cumin; pour stewed tomatoes and salsa over chicken. Simmer, uncovered, 15 minutes or until chicken is tender, turning once. With slotted spoon, remove chicken but reserve liquid in skillet. Shred chicken with two forks then return to skillet with green onion. Cook 2 minutes more or until most of liquid is absorbed. To serve, divide chicken mixture evenly down center of each tortilla, top with shredded lettuce, chopped tomato, and light/low fat cheese. Add cilantro; fold tortillas over filling. Serve immediately.

Perfect Pasta
By Nancy Schiemer

Ingredients:
One pound multigrain or whole wheat pasta
½ cup onion, chopped and sautéed.
¼ pound lean ground beef browned and drained.
2 spicy or sweet chicken sausage links, cooked and sliced
1 small container of part skim Ricotta cheese
One jar pasta sauce of your choice- I use 2 lb, 13 oz jar.
One two cup bag of low fat shredded mozzarella cheese

Instructions:
Cook ground beef until browned in med frying pan, drain.
Cook sausage thoroughly, chop up into pieces. These two
steps can be done the day before or another time and frozen
in packets to add when you are planning to make this dish.
Sauté onion, add meat and sausage and pasta sauce, warm
thoroughly. Cook pasta according to directions and drain,
and return to pot.
Add all ingredients except shredded mozzarella. Cheese into
large pot used to cook the pasta, mixing together. Pour into
two 8x8 or 9x9 pans, or one large 9x13 pan (prepared with
cooking spray).Top with mozzarella cheese. Cook at 350
degrees for about 30 min. or until bubbly. Cover last few
minutes if looking dry.

Potato and Collard Curry Soup
By Worcester Earn-A-Bike Organization

Makes: 10 Servings

Ingredients
2 medium onions
4 large cloves of garlic
8 red potatoes
2 bunches of collards (about 16 large leaves) or Kale
2 carrots
3 cups water
4 cups unsweetened soymilk
½ cup coconut milk
2 T tamari
3 T olive oil
1 t Jamaican curry
1 t Indian curry
2 t cilantro
¼ t red pepper
¼ t dry mustard
½ t rosemary
¼ t savory

Instructions:
Finely chop onions and garlic, add to large soup pot along with olive oil, simmer until soft. After about 5 minutes of simmering, add all the spices and the tamari, simmer another 2 minutes or so. Chop potatoes and carrots into bite-size pieces, add to soup pot when the onions and garlic are ready. Add the 3 cups of water. Bring to a strong simmer for about 10 minutes while preparing the collards. Cut the leaves away from the central stem, and chop finely into bite-size pieces. Add to the soup pot after potatoes and carrots have cooked for about 10 minutes. Continue simmering all ingredients until the potatoes, carrots and collards are all done. Add the soymilk and coconut milk, but do not let them boil. Let the soup sit for 10 minutes, stir and keep warm.

20 Minute Pasta Fagioli
By Luanne Monahan

Ingredients:
Water
Vegetable Oil Spray
1-2 Bay Leaves
Ditalini
Kidney Beans
Red Sauce
Salt
Black Pepper
Oregano
Chopped Onion/Chopped Garlic

Instructions:
Spray bottom of large, deep pot with vegetable oil spray. Pour in water and 1-2 bay leaves. Bring to a boil then reduce heat to medium/medium high. Add the ditalini, kidney beans, red sauce, salt, black pepper, oregano, and chopped onions/chopped garlic/garlic powder (sautéed in oil until browned). If adding lean beef or ground chicken/turkey, cook first and add along with the other ingredients. Serve with salad and a crusty whole grain or multigrain bread.

Healthy Burgers
By Sue Lasch

Ingredients:
1 lb. ground turkey or chicken
1/2 cup fresh mushrooms, chopped (can substitute with baby bellas)
1 cup fresh spinach, chopped fine
1 garlic clove, minced
1/2 cup reduced fat cheese
1-2 tbsp EVOO

Instructions:
Mix all of the above together and form into patties and grill, broil or pan fry till done. Serve mine on a bed of field greens with a slice of fresh avocado and tomato on top.

Grilled Turkey or Chicken Burgers
By Nancy Schiemer

Ingredients:
Lean Ground Turkey or Chicken
Italian Seasoning
Whole Wheat English Muffins
Low Fat Cheese

Instructions:
Preheat grill or other heat source. Prepare ground turkey or chicken into burger patties. Make sure to wash hands thoroughly after handling raw food. Place on the hot grill or pan. Sprinkle with Italian seasoning on first side. Reapply Italian seasoning when flipped over. Cook until inside is hot and no longer pink at all. Serve with low fat cheese on whole wheat English muffins or rolls. Add BBQ sauce if you'd like.

Marissa's Zucchini Pasta
By Marissa Bognanno

Makes: 2-4 servings

Ingredients:
2 medium zucchinis
2 tablespoons olive oil
1 clove garlic (whole)
½ pound penne rigate
crushed red pepper
salt + pepper

Instructions
Bring a large pot of salted water to a boil over high heat. Meanwhile, using a cheese grater, grate both zucchinis. Heat oil in a pan on medium heat and add the whole garlic clove. When it starts to sizzle, add in the zucchini and stir. Add salt (about 1 tsp) and crushed red pepper to taste. When the water is boiling, add the pasta and cook until tender but still firm to the bite, stirring occasionally, 8-10 minutes. Drain. Remove the garlic clove from the zucchini and check for additional seasonings. Toss with the pasta and add a few tablespoons of the pasta cooking liquid if necessary. Serve immediately with grated Parmesan cheese.

Mike's Lean Protein Pizza
By Michael J. Schiemer

Ingredients:
1 tsp honey
2 1/4 tsp active dry yeast
1 cup warm water
1 1/2 tsp salt
1 1/2 cups whole wheat flour
1/4 cup buckwheat flour
1/4 cup soy flour
4 tsp gluten
2 TBSP ground flaxseed
Tomato sauce
Fat Free shredded cheddar and mozzarella cheese

Instructions:
The preparation time is about an hour and the total time for this recipe is about 90 minutes. First, dissolve honey and yeast in warm water, let sit for about 7 minutes. Stir in salt, flours, ground flaxseed, and gluten. Knead for 5 minute place dough in bowl sprayed with cooking spray. Cover and let rise 45 minutes. Punch down and divide in half. Roll out and place on two 12 inch pizza pans sprayed with cooking spray. Preheat oven to 450 degrees and bake for 5 minutes. Remove from oven and add sufficient tomato sauce and plenty of fat free shredded cheese. I usually also add roasted or grilled vegetables or chicken. Bake for 15 minutes and enjoy this filling yet guilt-free pizza!

Spinach pie
By Nancy Schiemer

Ingredients:
One prepared deep crust pie shell- can be frozen
One package of frozen chopped spinach, thawed and drained
One pint part skim ricotta cheese
½ onion chopped fine
½ tsp minced garlic
Sea salt and pepper to taste (optional)
Low fat cheese, 3 large 5x5" slices
One egg or egg beater

Instructions:
Combine spinach (drained) with ricotta, onion, garlic and
egg (salt and pepper) and mix well. Pour mixture into pie
shell. Top with cheese. You can also sprinkle some
parmesan cheese on top too! Bake at 350 degrees until the
top is golden brown, about 30-40 min.

Zucchini Bread
By Chef Corin Szostek

Ingredients:
3 eggs
1 c extra virgin olive oil
1/4 c sugar or Splenda
1/2 c Splenda brown sugar mix
2 tsp. baking soda
1 tsp salt (optional)
1/4 tsp. baking powder
2 tsp. cinnamon

Instructions:
Blend the first 4 ingredients together. Then blend the rest of the
ingredients together. Then add along 2 cups grated zucchini (par
boil). Bake for 1 hour at 350 degrees F.

Lentil and Kale Soup
By Joanne Koch

Makes: 6

Ingredients:
1 lb green lentils
2 t sea salt
1/2 c olive oil
1 bay leaf
1 cup chopped onion
2 stalks celery, chopped
2 carrots chopped
2 garlic gloves mashed
1 bunch kale, thinly sliced
1 pound tomatoes, peeled and chopped
3 16 oz cans of chicken broth
1 bunch fresh parsley, chopped 1/4 t black pepper, freshly ground

Instructions:
Wash and drain lentils and place in soup pot. Cover with water and add 1 t salt. Bring to boil and cook for 5 minutes. Drain and rinse. Heat olive oil in soup pot with bay leaf. Add onions, celery, carrots, and garlic. Add kale and simmer for 5 minutes. Stir in tomatoes. Add chicken stock, lentils, and remaining sea salt. Blend ingredients and bring to a boil. Reduce heat and simmer for 15 minutes. Add chopped parsley and pepper. Divide into bowls and add freshly grated parmesan cheese, parsley and a few drops of olive oil.

Breaded Chicken In The Oven
By Nancy Schiemer

Ingredients:
Two pounds boneless chicken breasts
One large egg, scrambled + two tablespoons of water
Italian seasoned bread crumbs
Flour
Garlic powder
Italian seasoning
Parmesan cheese
Chicken broth, canned or use a bouillon cube

Instructions:
Preheat oven to 350 degrees. Mix Italian bread crumbs with garlic powder to your taste, add Italian seasoning, about two shakes. Add parmesan cheese, about two tablespoons. Set aside this mixture in a large flat bowl or plate. Place chicken breasts in between wax paper and pound until flattened. Dredge through flour, dip in egg mixture and then turn into and cover with bread crumbs Place into a lightly greased 13 x 9" pan. Cook at 350 degrees. Pour in chicken broth after 20 min. to keep moist as it cooks. Cook at 350 degrees until no longer pink in the center, about 30-40 min.

Pepperoni e Patate (Vegan)
By Amanda Baldi

Instructions:
Julienned red and green peppers
Peeled and thinly sliced potatoes
Olive oil
Garlic
Rosemary
Chopped onion

Instructions:
Heat two skillets. The bottoms should be coated with olive oil. In one skillet, put a few cloves of garlic. In the other, put about a handful of chopped onion just for taste. The oil is ready when bubbles form around a toothpick's point. Once the oil is heated, put the peppers into the garlic skillet and put the potatoes into the onion skillet. Stir the peppers to prevent burning. Flip the potatoes to prevent burning. Once the peppers are soft and the potatoes are saturated, put them into the same skillet and add rosemary to taste. Over medium heat, mix them around a bit.

Caesar Salad
By Chef Corin Szostek

Makes: 4 to 6 servings

Ingredients:
For Croutons:
 2 tablespoons unsalted margarine/vegetable oil spread
2 tablespoons extra virgin olive oil
1 eight-ten ounce loaf of bread, crusts removed, cut into 3/4 inch pieces
1 teaspoon salt
1/4 teaspoon ground cayenne pepper

1/2 teaspoons freshly ground black pepper
For Salad:
2 cloves garlic
4 anchovy filets (optional)
1 teaspoon salt
1 tablespoon freshly squeezed lemon juice
1 teaspoon Worcestershire sauce
1 teaspoon Dijon mustard
1 large egg yolk
1/3 cup extra virgin olive oil
2 ten ounce heads romaine lettuce, outer leaves discarded, inner leaves washed and dried
1 cup freshly grated parmesan or Romano cheese, or 2 1/2 ounces shaved

Instructions:
If you prefer not to use the raw yolk in this recipe, substitute one tablespoon of store bought mayonnaise. The croutons are best made close to serving time as possible. Heat oven to 450 degrees. Combine butter and olive oil in a large bowl. Add bread cubes and toss until coated. Sprinkle salt, cayenne pepper and black pepper; toss until evenly coated. Spread bread in a single layer on an 11" x 7" baking sheet. Bake until croutons are golden, about 10 minutes. Set aside until needed. Place garlic, anchovy fillets and salt in a large wooden salad bowl. Using two dinner forks, mash the garlic and anchovies into a paste. Using one fork, whisk in pepper, lemon juice, Worcestershire sauce, Dijon mustard and egg yolk. Using the fork, whisk in the olive oil. Chop romaine leaves into 1 to 1 1/2 inch pieces. Add croutons, romaine and cheese to the bowl, and toss well. If you wish, grate extra cheese over the top. Serve immediately. To make a version of this dressing that you can store, simply mince garlic and anchovies, and place with remaining ingredients in a jar. Screw the lid on the jar tightly, and shake to combine. Shake the jar before each use. Store, refrigerated, up to 4 days, If you wish to make this a main meal you can add grilled chicken, grilled steak, shrimp or scallops.

Quiche For One
By Nancy Schiemer

Ingredients:
Small loaf pan ~ 3" x 5"
Two egg whites, or two egg substitutes or two scrambled eggs
Hand full of raw spinach, ripped into small pieces
Slice block of reduced fat jalapeño cheese- about 4 slices, or enough to top loaf pan
Canola oil cooking spray
One slice of whole wheat/multigrain bread or whole wheat English muffin, uncooked

Instructions:
Preheat toaster oven or regular oven to 350 degrees. Spray pan with canola oil spray. Tear off pieces of bread, put ½ into the pan. Add spinach on top of bread. Add the rest of the bread. Pour egg mixture over entire bread/ spinach mixture. Top with cheese slices. Cook about 25 min. or until brown on top. This takes about two minutes to prepare, then you could cook it while showering; then bring it to work and eat it for breakfast or lunch.

Additional Options to Add:
Broccoli in small pieces, blanched first, ½ cup
Sliced cooked onion, ¼ cup
Triple the recipe, cook it in a large loaf pan (cook it longer though) and eat it three times that week, or cook it in three pans and you are ready for several meals.

Broccoli Casserole:
By Chef Corin Szostek

Ingredients:
156 oz. pkg. of frozen cut broccoli
1 can of low sodium cream of mushroom soup
8 oz low fat or fat free cheddar cheese cup up
1/2- 3/4 package of seasoned croutons

Instructions:
Mix all ingredients together thoroughly and add to a large casserole dish. Bake at 350 degrees until bubbly (Approximately 45 minutes)

Zucchini Casserole
By Chef Corin Szostek

Ingredients:
1-2 zucchinis sliced + par boil 8 min (drain well)
1 can of low sodium cream of mushroom soup
1/2 c fat free or low fat grated cheddar cheese
1/4 cup low fat sour cream
1 large carrot grated
1 medium onion chopped fine
mix together
1 stick vegetable oil spread/margarine
8 oz pkg. stuffing mix

Instructions:
In a 9" x 13" casserole dish put 1/2 stuffing mix on bottom. Mix zucchini with separate bowl mixture carefully. Spoon into casserole and put rest of stuffing mix on top. Bake at 325 degrees for approximately 45 minutes.

Sugo All'Ascollana / Sugo Magro (Pescatarian)
By Amanda Baldi

Ingredients:
15 Anchovies
4-5 Cups Green Olives
4 tbsp Olive Oil
3-4 Minced Cloves of Garlic
3 Jars Tomato Sauce
Salt and Pepper
1.5 Cans of Tuna
Whole Wheat Spaghetti
Cilantro

Instructions:
Rinse about 15 anchovies in water and clean them of spines and tails. You will need about 4 or 5 cups of green olives. Pit them by cutting the skins off with a paring knife. Try not to mince the skin as you go. Heat olive oil (4 tbsp) in a skillet with 3-4 minced cloves of garlic. Add fresh cilantro to the skillet. Add anchovies to the skillet and stir them. They should break up into little pieces. Add crushed red pepper to taste, and the pitted olives. Let simmer for about 10-15 minutes. For this recipe, we used homemade tomato pulp which we strained of water. If using store-bought tomato sauce, my guess is that you won't have to do this. We added probably the equivalent of 3 jars of store-bought sauce. Sprinkle on a bunch of salt, and add black pepper to taste. Boil over high heat for 10 minutes or so. Boiling for a long time over low heat causes tomatoes to lose their "properties" and flavor. Cook tomatoes over high heat for a short time. Add about a can and 1/2 of Tonno tuna fish, and let it heat through. Serve hot over spaghetti.

Boiled Potatoes (Vegan)
By Amanda Baldi

Ingredients:
3 Potatoes
Pot of Water
Vinegar
Salt and pepper
Olive Oil
Chives

Instructions:
Clean a few potatoes and put them in a pot of cold water. Set it on the stove to boil. When boiled through, pick out the potatoes (with a spoon). Once cool enough to handle, peel off the skin. Cut potatoes short-ways; they should break up easily. Douse with a bit of vinegar, add salt and pepper. Add some tasty olive oil to taste (the more the better in my estimation), and sprinkle with chives.

Turkey Meatballs
By Nancy Schiemer

Ingredients:
One pound lean ground turkey or chicken.
½ teaspoon Italian seasoning.
Two shakes garlic powder
½ cup water
½ cup breadcrumbs
Salt and pepper to taste

Instructions:
Preheat oven to 350 degrees. Mix all together in a bowl. Roll into small meatballs. Bake in oven for about 20 min. turning once at 10 minutes. Check to see that center is hot and cooked through. Serve with any whole wheat or whole grain pasta and sauce. OR use in whole wheat rolls for meatball sandwiches with sauce. Top with part skim mozzarella cheese and broil until cheese is bubbly.

Sautéed Zucchini and Potatoes (Vegan)
By Amanda Baldi

Ingredients:
Olive oil
1/2 onion, chopped
4-6 zucchini, chopped
Salt
5 med potatoes, peeled and chopped
Mint
Basil

Instructions:
In a large, deep skillet, heat a substantial amount of olive oil, maybe 1/4" deep. When the oil is hot, add the onions and sauté slowly until they are golden brown. Do not burn. Olive oil is adequately heated if, when a toothpick is inserted, bubbles form around it. Add the zucchini and salt. The salt should be distributed throughout the skillet on the zucchini to draw out the water. Cover and let simmer for 20 minutes. In a separate large skillet, heat 1/4" of olive oil. Add potatoes at low heat. Stir to keep from burning. When they have been cooked through (aka: olive oil has soaked all the way through), and they are a light golden brown, add the potatoes to the zucchini mixture. Cover, simmer 5 minutes. Add chopped fresh mint and basil. Simmer 5 minutes.

Garden Macaroni Salad
By Chef Corin Szostek

Ingredients:
1 cup diced carrots
3/4 cups low fat or fat free mayonnaise
1/4 tsp. basil
8 oz. Whole Wheat elbow macaroni-cooked
1 cup celery
1/4 cup diced green peppers
2 tsp. sliced onions
1/2 cup dill pickle juice

Instructions:
Stir ingredients together thoroughly, cover, and chill until served.

Taco Salad
By Chef Corin Szostek

Ingredients:
1/4 lb. lean ground beef or turkey
1 can kidney beans
1/4 c. onions, chopped
1/2 head lettuce, shredded
1 green pepper, coarsely chopped
1 tomato, seeded and chopped
2 cups multi grain corn chips or healthy pita chips
1 cup low-fat or fat free shredded cheese

Instructions:
In a small skillet brown the meat thoroughly: stir in the beans and heat through. Place corn chips in a bowl. Spoon in the meat mixture. Top with onions, lettuce, green pepper, tomato and cheese. Serve with taco sauce or salsa.

Easy Sloppy Joes
By Chef Corin Szostek

Ingredients:
1/2 lb. lean ground beef, turkey, or chicken
1/4 c Ketchup
2 TBSP minced onion
1/2 can chicken gumbo soup

Instructions:
Brown ground beef. Stir in ketchup, onion and chicken gumbo soup. Cover and simmer for 10-15 minutes, stirring occasionally. Serve on whole wheat hamburger buns.

Chicken Cacciatore
By Chef Corin Szostek

Ingredients:
2-3 lbs. chicken breast
2 tbsp whole wheat flour
2 tbsp. chopped onions
1/2 cup tomato paste
3/4 cup chicken broth or water
1/8 tsp. thyme
1/2 tsp. basil
1 cup mushrooms
1 tsp. salt
Green pepper (optional)
1/2 cup dry white wine (optional)

Instructions:
Cut chicken into individual pieces. Dredge with flour and sauté until brown in olive oil. Add remaining ingredients and simmer covered for 1 hour or until tender. Best served with brown rice, quinoa, or whole grain pasta

Lean Greek Lasagna
By Chef Mark Brambilla

Ingredients:
2 sticks of margarine
1 1/2 lbs of ground meat
1 onion chopped fine
1 can tomato puree
1 bay leaf
1 tsp cinnamon
1 lb brown rice pasta shells
3 cups parmesan cheese
3/4 cup flour
3 1/2 cups rice milk
5 eggs

Instructions:
Melt margarine, add hamburger and onion. Cook. Add
tomato puree, bay leave, and cinnamon. Cook macaroni
shells. Place cooked pasta in pan. Top with meat mixture.
For topping: mix 1 stick of margarine and flour. Heat rice
milk, add little to flour mixture. Then add flour mixture to
milk. Thicken, and add eggs until thickens. Pour over eat
and pasta. Bake for 1 hour. You may add spinach to meat
mixture if desired.

Guglielmo Family Homemade Tortellini
By Chef Corin Szostek

Ingredients:
Full bag of whole wheat flour
3 Eggs
Lean Ground Meat
Garlic
Parmesan Cheese
Tomato Sauce

Cooking Utensils:
Pasta making machine

Instructions:
Cook meat in oven and then grind it up in food processor. We use pork and buy a pork roast and cook the roast before grinding. When cooking in oven and/or when grinding add garlic for flavor. Then put ground meat in a medium to big sized bowl. Then combine eggs and flour in food processor to make dough. Make sure the dough isn't too sticky and sticks just enough. Then put dough in a medium to big sized bowl. Then take small to medium amount of the dough and run it through the pasta machine, cutting with a knife if necessary. Then after it is rolled through the pasta machine and is all stretched and flat place it either on the board or directly onto the table. Make sure the table or board is lightly floured. Then cut the dough length with down and across with the pizza cutter making little to medium sized squares. Then take small amounts of the ground meat and out it in the squares you just cut. Make sure you don't put too much because you don't want more meat then dough and then it won't fold. Then take the squares filled with meat and fold them diagonally to fold to make sure they are closed. Then on a platter or plate put the finished ones. Stick them in the freezer for a fast freeze and you make as many as you can. Then when all are made you can put them into zip lock bags, freezer bags, or Tupperware containers to keep them frozen until ready to cook. Cook them in chicken soup broth. Sprinkle grated cheese on it and top with a tomato sauce.

Chicken Diane
By Chef Corin Szostek

Ingredients:

6 boneless, skinless chicken thighs or breast halves
1 medium onion, chopped fine
1/3 cup fresh parsley
1/4 cup dry sherry
1 tablespoon Worcestershire sauce
1 tablespoon Dijon-style mustard
fresh or canned mushrooms

Instructions:

In a large skillet, add the chicken and cook, turning frequently until lightly browned on all sides and, when pierced with a fork, juices run clear. Remove chicken to a plate and keep warm. In the same skillet, heat remaining butter. Add onion and sauté until translucent, about 2 minutes or less. Reduce heat and add remaining ingredients, except chicken. Cook, stirring occasionally, until heated through. Return chicken to skillet and turn to coat with sauce.

Hearty Post-Workout Chili
By Chef Mark Brambilla

Ingredients:
1/2 cup red wine
2 T. cumin
16 oz black beans
2 large jalapenos chopped
1/3 cup chili powder
28 oz whole tomatoes chopped with reserved liquid
2 lbs pork butt in 1 inch cubes
1 lb beef stew meat in 1 inch cubes
3 garlic cloves chopped
2 green bell peppers chopped
2 onions chopped
3 T. olive oil

Instructions:
Heat oil, and sauté onions, peppers, and garlic. Sauté until tender for 14 minutes. Transfer mixture to a plate. Add beef and pork and sauté 10 minutes or no longer pink. Return onion mixture, add tomatoes with liquid, add chili powder, jalapeños, and cumin. Season with salt and pepper if desired. Cover and simmer 1 hour until meat is tender. Add black beans and red wine to chili. Simmer until thicken and tender. About 30 minutes. Adjust seasoning. Ladle into bowls with garnish of choice.

Corin's Chili
By Chef Corin Szostek

Ingredients:
1 lb. lean ground beef or turkey
1 large onion chopped
1   8 oz tomato sauce
1 tsp. salt
1 bay leaf
1 green pepper chopped
1 can tomatoes (2 cups)
1   lb kidney beans
2 tsp. chili powder

Instructions:
Brown meat, onions, and peppers. Add rest of ingredients
and simmer for 1 hour.

Cucumber Soup
By Marissa Bognanno

Ingredients:
1 large cucumber
1/4 cup light sour cream
Fresh mint
1/2 tsp kosher salt
1/2 tsp black pepper
Pinch cayenne

Instructions:
Roughly chop the cucumber and mix with several sprigs of
the fresh mint, salt, pepper and cayenne. Drop into a
blender. Scoop in the sour cream. Blend until creamy and
velvety. Serve with crusty bread and brie!

Quinoa Salad (Gluten-Free)
By Paula Pelavin

Ingredients:
1 cup quinoa cooked
2 tomatoes (or a handful of cherry tomatoes)
1/2 bell pepper (red, yellow, or orange)
1/2 cucumber
1 or 2 cloves garlic diced
1 bunch parsley
1 handful of basil leaves
Chickpeas (optional)

Dressing:
2 Tbsp olive oil
2 Tbsp lemon juice
1. Tbsp white balsamic vinegar or other light vinegar
salt and pepper

Instructions:
For the veggies take out seeds from all and do a fine chop.
Rough chop all of the herbs. Mix salad thoroughly and add
dressing liberally.

Sherried Beef-Onion Bake
By Katie Koch

Makes: 4 Servings

Ingredients:
2 Tbsp vegetable oil spread
2 Tbsp whole wheat flour
Dash of pepper
1 Cup water
¼ Cup Dry Sherry or White Wine
2 TSP instant beef bouillon granules
1 pound Lean Beef cut into 1 inch cubes
¼ TSP kitchen bouquet
2 Large Onions cut into wedges
¾ Cup multigrain/whole grain croutons
1/3 Cup Low Fat Swiss Cheese Shredded
2 TBSP grated Parmesan Cheese
Snipped Parsley (optional)

Instructions:
(Assembling time is about 25 minutes. Cooking time is about 2 hours) In a medium saucepan melt butter. Stir in flour and pepper. Add water, sherry, and bouillon granules to saucepan. Cook and stir until mixture is thickened and bubbly. Cook and stir for 1 minute more. Remove from heat. Stir in beef cubes and kitchen bouquet. Place onion wedges in a ½ qt casserole dish, spoon the meat mixture atop. Cover casserole and bake in 375 degrees oven for 105-120 minutes. Arrange croutons on top and sprinkle parmesan and Swiss Cheese. Cook uncovered for 5-10 more minutes and serve.

Chicken and Stuffing Bake
By Katie Koch

Ingredients:
6 skinless boneless chicken breast halves
1 can low fat cream of mushroom soup
1/3 cup skim milk
1 tsp chopped parsley
Stuffing mix (I use 2 cups Pepperidge Farm)
 2/3 cup water
2 tbsp Smart Balance butter.

Instructions:
Heat oven to 400 degrees. Put stuffing across center of 2 qt baking dish. Arrange chicken on each side, combine soup, milk and parsley and pour over chicken. Cover with foil and bake ¾ hour.

Crunchy Tangy Orange Oven/Fried Chicken
By Catherine Lawrie

Ingredients:
1 1/2 pounds of boneless skinless chicken breasts
1/2 cup panko bread crumbs
1/2 cup wheat germ
1 cup of orange juice
1 cup of plain yogurt

Instructions:
Preheat oven to 425. Bake for 35 minutes. Marinade chicken in orange juice for several hours in fridge, Pat dry. Spread yogurt evenly over chicken breasts. Mix bread crumbs and wheat germ together in a shallow dish or sealable bag. Dredge chicken in mixture covering evenly. Place chicken breast in a glass baking dish sprayed with non stick spray. Goes great with brown rice! For kids you can make healthy nuggets this way too- just cut into bite size pieces

Lazy-Ana (Lasagna)
By Mirella Santucci

Ingredients:
1 lbs. of whole- wheat pasta-spiral or ziti
1 lbs. of Italian seasoned ground Turkey meat
2 cups of tomato sauce
1 small white onion
6 tbsp of extra virgin olive oil
1 pkg. of white cap mushrooms
½ cup of 2% milk mozzarella
¼ cup of grated parmesan cheese
¾ of small peas-optional

Instructions:
This is a great dish because it's quick- easy and tastes even better the next day. All you do is sauté your leftovers, in a non-stick skillet with ¼ cup of water, for 3-4 minutes. Then add ¼ tsp. crush red pepper flakes; drizzle extra virgin olive oil & sprinkle parmesan cheese & your done –Delicious! Prepare spiral whole-wheat pasta according to the directions. Drain pasta & water from the pasta pot: place cooked pasta back into the pasta pot and cover to keep warm & set aside. In a nonstick skillet sauté Italian seasoned ground turkey meat with olive oil. Cook the turkey meat for 5-10 minutes than gradually adding the onions, peas & mushrooms. Continue cooking until onions become opaque & meat is fully cooked. While the meat mixture is still hot, immediately add it to the cooked pasta in the pasta pot. Warm up the 2 cups of tomato sauce in the skillet than add to the pasta. Fold in ½ the mozzarella cheese and mix; top the pasta with the parmesan cheese & cover. Let stand for about 5 minutes in the pot before serving.

Shrimp Scampi
By Sue Lasch

Ingredients:
1 lb shrimp, fresh or frozen, peeled and deveined
1/4 cup fresh lemon juice
2-3 tbsp fresh chopped parsley
4 garlic cloves, chopped
3 tbsp EVOO or trans-fat free margarine
Salt and pepper

Instructions:
Heat EVOO/margarine in frying pan over medium heat, add garlic, simmer 1-2 minutes then add shrimp. Toss shrimp to coat with olive oil/garlic mixture. Add lemon juice and parsley and cook shrimp till done, 4-5 minutes. Avoid overcooking as it makes the shrimp tough. Remove from heat and season with salt and pepper. Serve over whole wheat pasta or steamed asparagus.

Crispy Chicken
By Michael J. Schiemer

Ingredients:
2 Eggs
2 Chicken Breasts
1-2 Cups Light or Whole Grain Bread Crumbs
Tomatoe Sauce
Fat Free Cheese
Canola Oil or Canola Oil Spray

Instructions:
Have a frying pan on medium-high, a bowl with 2 beaten eggs, and a bowl with the bread crumbs. After cutting off any excess fat from the chicken breasts, coat chicken breast with egg, then bread crumbs, then add to the frying pan after it has been coated or sprayed with canola oil. Fry until chicken is cooked through and bread crumbs are crispy. Top with tomato sauce and cheese.

Chicken or Steak Quesadillas
By Michael J. Schiemer

Ingredients:
Whole wheat tortillas, soft
Low Fat Monterey, Cheddar, and/or Mozzarella Cheese
Chicken breasts grilled or grilled steak like a London broil cut
Canola Oil
Salsa (optional)
Fat Free Sour Cream (optional)
Grilled Onions
Red Peppers
Grilled Peppers

Instructions:
Chop up chicken or steak into ½ to 1" pieces. Pour canola oil into 10-12" frying pan, heat oil on medium. On the counter, place chicken pieces on ½ of a tortilla, sprinkle with a handful of shredded cheese, then fold it over. Repeat with another tortilla. Place both tortillas in the pan, facing each other with the folded edges. Heat until golden and flip to the other sides. Repeat until brown and keep warm in oven or toaster oven. Continue making them until you have used up your chicken and steak. Refrigerate extra quesadillas for later.

Grilled Shrimp Kabob
By Nancy Schiemer

Ingredients:
2 TBSP lemon juice
2 TBSP lime juice
2 TBSP plain or flavored garlic oil
1/4 tsp ground cinnamon
1/4 tsp paprika
1 TBSP chopped fresh cilantro
1 1/4 pound large peeled shrimp (16-20 count)
Lemon wedges
Wooden skewers (soaked in water for 30 minutes)

Instructions:
Combine all ingredients except shrimp and lemon wedges.
Prepare or heat grill to high heat. Toss shrimp with marinade
in a large bowl or plastic bag and marinate for about 10
minutes. The texture of shrimp will change if left in
marinade too long. Place shrimp on wooden skewers
alternating with fresh lemon wedges and grill, basting
frequently with marinade, until shrimp turns pink (about 2
minutes per side). Serve and enjoy!

Salmon Fillets For Four with Marinade/Sauce
By Nancy Schiemer

Ingredients:
2 Tbsp Dijon mustard
3 Tbsp Soy sauce
6 Tbsp Olive oil
½ tsp. minced garlic
2 lbs Salmon fillets

Instructions:
While the grill is heating (or broiler), lay the salmon skin side down on a cutting board and cut it cross-wide into 4 equal pieces. Whisk together the mustard, soy sauce, olive oil, and garlic in a small bowl. Drizzle half of the marinade onto the salmon and allow it to sit for 10 minutes. Just drizzle, don't overdo the amount as it tends to flame up if it's too much. Save the other half of the marinade you haven't used. Place salmon skin side down on the grill. Discard the marinade the fish was sitting in. Grill 4-5 minutes depending on the thickness of the fish. Turn carefully with a wide spatula and grill for another 4-5 minutes. The salmon will be slightly raw in the center, but don't worry, it will keep cooking as it sits. Transfer the fish to a flat plate, skin side down and spoon the reserved marinade on top. This marinade makes the dish! Allow the fish to rest for 10 minutes. Remove the skin and serve warm, at room temp or chilled.

Orechiette with Shrimp (Pescatarian)
By Amanda Baldi

Ingredients:
Whole Wheat Pasta
Shrimp
Olive Oil
Fresh Thyme, Parsley, Rosemary

Instructions:
Boil the pasta. When it is al dente, plate it and top with shrimp, olive oil, and chopped aromatic herbs and salt to taste. Voila! Serve while the pasta is still hot. This is a typical dish of Puglia. It is simple, delicious, and healthy.

Healthier Meatballs
By Chef Corin Szostek

Ingredients:
1 pound of lean ground beef, chicken, pork, or turkey
half chopped onion
pepper
parsley flakes
bread crumbs
Skim Milk
1 egg
¼ Cup Wheat Germ (optional)

Instructions:
Mix ingredients thoroughly. Shape into balls, spread out on a tray. Place in the oven and cook thoroughly. Serve with whole grain pasta and tomato sauce.

Salmon Cakes:
By Chef Mark Brambilla

Makes: 4 Servings

Ingredients:
2 1/2 cups salmon fresh shredded
1/2 cups fresh bread crumbs
1 T. Dijon mustard
1 tsp lime
1 large egg
1 cup pistachio nuts coarse ground
3 T. olive oil

Instructions:
Combine salmon, bread crumbs, Dijon mustard, and lime.
Stir in the egg and mix. Form salmon into patties and press
on the ground pistachio nuts. Chill for 30 minutes to 2
hours. Pan-fry and serve with lime wedge.

Creamed Corn With Canadian Bacon
By Chef Mark Brambilla and Brie

Ingredients:
2-4 fresh corn cooked and scraped off cob
2 T. flour
1 1/2 cup fat free milk
2 tsp. sugar
1/4 tsp salt
2 tsp butter
1/4 diced ham
1/4 finely diced onion
1 garlic clove minced

Instructions:
Combine 1 cup corn, flour, milk, sugar, salt. Process until smooth. Melt butter, Add ham, onion, and garlic. Cook 3 minutes until browned. Add pureed corn and rest of corn. Cook for 12 minutes or until thickened.

Mike's Simple Chicken Salad
By Michael J. Schiemer

Ingredients:
2-3 Cups Spinach Salad
6 oz Grilled Chicken Strips
½ Cup Fat Free Cheese
½ Cup Cherry Tomatoes
2 TBSP Olive Oil + Garlic

Instructions:
Start with plenty of spinach salad for extra antioxidants. Add the grilled chicken strips or cubes, then cheese, cherry tomatoes, and top with olive oil mixed with garlic or garlic powder.

Quick Snack Recipes

English Muffin Pizzas
By Michael J. Schiemer

Ingredients:
2 Whole Wheat English Muffins
2 Tbsp Tomato Sauce
1 Cup Fat Free Shredded Cheese
Italian Seasonings

Instructions:
Slice English muffins if they aren't already and then toast them until crispy in a toaster oven or toaster. Spread tomato sauce evenly on each side and then top liberally with fat free shredded cheddar cheese. Add Italian spices for a little extra flavor and enjoy a very healthy, quick, and delicious snack.

Home-Made Hummus
By Nancy Schiemer

Makes: 5 Servings

Ingredients:
1 can chick peas
3 tbsp tahini
1 clove garlic, chopped fine
1 tsp salt,
1 lemon's juice
¼ cup chick pea juice

Instructions:
Drain chick peas saving ¼ cup as above for the recipe. Place in blender with other ingredients. Blend until smooth, extra lemon and or garlic can be added for flavor.

Home-Made Tomato Sauce
By Chef Corin Szostek

Ingredients:
2 large cans of ground peeled tomatoes (28 ounces each)
1 can 6 oz tomato paste
1 pound lean ground beef
1 package lean Italian, chicken, or turkey sausages
1 large onion
2 cloves of garlic
1/3 cup extra virgin olive oil
Parsley flakes
Pepper

Instructions:
Chop onion and garlic. Add to olive oil in large sauce pan.
Sauté with sausages and meatballs for about 5 minutes. Add
tomatoes. Sprinkle pepper to taste and parsley flakes. Cook
on low with a cover for about 20 minutes. Add paste. Stir
frequently during the 3 hours of cooking. Cook on low and
add more pepper and parsley to taste.

Edamame Feta Dip
By Chef Mark Brambilla

Ingredients:
2 cups shelled edamames
3 cloves garlic
1/2 cup feta cheese
2 1/2 T. fresh lemon
2 T. olive oil
Salt and pepper

Instructions:
Boil and cook edamames until completely tender. Reserve
1/2 of cooking liquid. Puree all and serve chilled with baked
pita chips.

Spicy Sweet Humus
By Chef Corin Szostek

Ingredients:
1 (15 ounce) can chickpeas, drained
1 (4 oz jar roasted red peppers
3 tablespoons lemon juice
1 1/2 tablespoons tahini
1 clove garlic minced
1/2 teaspoon ground cumin
1/2 teaspoon cayenne pepper
1/4 teaspoon salt
1 tablespoon chopped fresh parsley

Instructions:
Puree the chickpeas, red peppers, lemon juice, tahini, garlic, cumin, cayenne and salt. Process, using long pulses, until the mixture is fairly smooth, and slightly fluffy. Scrape the mixture off the sides of the food processor or blender in between pulses. Transfer to a serving bowl and refrigerate for at least 1 hour. The hummus can be made up to 3 days ahead and refrigerated. Sprinkle the hummus with chopped parsley before serving.

Approximate Nutritional Content: (Per Serving) Calories: 25, Total Fat: 2 g, Cholesterol: 0 mg, Sodium: 250 mg, Total Carbohydrate: 2 g, Dietary Fiber: 0.5 g, Protein: 1 g

Home-Made Granola
By Christine Van Zadelhoff

Ingredients:
6 Cups Old Fashioned Oats
1 Cup Almonds or other nuts
¼ Cup Sunflower Seeds
1/3 Cup flaxseed meal and/or wheat germ
1 tsp Cinnamon
3 Egg Whites
1 tsp salt (or salt substitute)
1 Cup Honey, Agave Nectar, or Molasses
1/3 Cup Extra Virgin Olive Oil
1 Cup Dried Fruits, chopped

Instructions:
Preheat the oven to 350 degrees. Combine oats, nuts, seeds, flaxseed/wheat germ, and cinnamon in a large bowl. In another bowl, whisk the egg whites and salt until frothy. Whisk in your choice of sweetener and olive oil. Add the wet ingredients to the dry ingredients and stir until oats are evenly coated. Transfer mixture to two rimmed baking sheets and spread flat. Bake for 20 minutes then gently flip with spatula, moving granola from the outer edges to the center of the sheet. Continue to cook for about 10 minutes or until golden. Cool completely on the pan then transfer to a bowl and gently stir in the dried fruit.

Lisa's Light Pizza
By Lisa Gardiner

Makes: 1 Serving

Ingredients:
1 round piece of Syrian bread.
Spread with any classic or flavored humus of choice.
Cover with a thin layer of tabouli.
Sprinkle with feta cheese.
Eat room temp or cold.

Instructions:
This recipe only takes 2 minutes to make. Cut it like a pizza.
Add toppings such as olives, diced peppers, etc.

Sautéed Garlic Spinach
By Nancy Schiemer

Makes: 4 Servings

Ingredients:
Large bag spinach, raw, washed.
½ teaspoon of garlic (more if you love garlic)
One to two tablespoons of Olive Oil
Salt to taste

Instructions:
In a large pot on stove on medium heat, sauté garlic in oil.
After garlic is fragrant, add spinach to pot and lower heat to
low setting. Cook and stir with tongs until all spinach has
been cooked down to soft cooked spinach.

Apple Sandwiches w/ Granola/Peanut Butter
By Chef Corin Szostek

Makes: 2 Servings

Ingredients:
2 small apples, cored and cut crosswise into 1/2 inch thick rounds
1 teaspoon lemon juice (optional)
3 tablespoons natural peanut butter
2 tablespoons semisweet or dark chocolate chips
3 tablespoons granola

Instructions:
If you won't be eating these tasty treats right away, start by brushing the apples slices with lemon juice to keep them from turning brown. Spread one side of half of the apple slices with peanut butter, the other side sprinkle with chocolate chips and granola. Top with remaining apple slices,
pressing down gently to make the sandwiches. Transfer to napkins or plates and serve.

Approximate Nutritional Content: Serving Size: 7 oz/192g, 300 calories (150 from fat), 16g total fat, 4.5g saturated fat, 0mg cholesterol, 115mg sodium, 36g total carbohydrate (6g dietary fiber, 25 g sugar), 8g protein.

(Turkey) Pepperoni Pizza Dip
By Chef Corin Szostek

Ingredients:
1 8 oz. Pk. Low Fat Cream Cheese
1/2 cup low fat dairy sour cream
1/8 tsp. garlic powder
1 tsp. oregano
1/8 tsp. crushed red pepper
1/2 cup pizza sauce
1/2 cup chopped or turkey pepperoni
1/4 cup sliced green onion
1/2 cup shredded low-fat mozzarella cheese

Instructions:
In a small mixing bowl beat together cream cheese, sour cream, oregano, garlic powder and red pepper. Spread evenly in 9 or 10 inch pie plate. Spread pizza sauce over the top. Sprinkle with pepperoni, green onion and green pepper. Bake in a 350 degree oven for 10 minutes. Top with mozzarella: bake 5 minutes more or until cheese is melted and mixture is heated through.

Cinnamon Toast
By Michael J. Schiemer

Ingredients:
2 Slices 12 Grain Bread
Margarine
Cinnamon
Splenda

Instructions:
Toast bread and spread margarine. Add cinnamon and pour small amounts of Splenda powder to make this sweet and cinnamon treat. It may not be the healthiest snack ever, but it's better for you than the cereal and better than the white bread and table sugar original.

Chocolate Peanut Butter Oatmeal Crisp
By Michael J. Schiemer

Makes: About 15 Servings

Ingredients:
1 lb Jar of Natural Peanut Butter
Dymatize 12 Hour Chocolate Protein Powder
100% Rolled Oats

Cooking Utensils:
Toaster Oven
Spoon

Instructions:
Open up your jar of natural peanut butter and mix any oil separation into the peanut butter. Eat a few scoops of the peanut butter to make room at the top for the additional ingredients. Add 1/3 to ½ of a scoop of chocolate whey protein powder. Add the oats, stir, and spoon this delicious and nutritious mixture into your mouth. Add more oats and protein powder as needed for the whole jar of peanut butter. I personally only like oats that are toasted and crunchy so I do just that. Add 1-2 cups of oats onto a metal toaster oven tray, cook in toaster oven until slightly browned and crispy, and then add them to the peanut butter. Save extra toasted oats in a bag after they have cooled down to add later.

Fruit Salad with Maraschino Liquer (Vegan)

By Amanda Baldi

Ingredients:
2 Pears, chopped
2 Kiwis, chopped
2 Peaches, chopped
2 Bananas, chopped
3 tbsp Maraschino liqueur

Instructions:
Chop all of the above-mentioned fruit into very small pieces. Add liqueur, evenly distributing it over the fruit. This may be served, also, over yogurt.

Crab Meat Dip

By Chef Corin Szostek

Ingredients:
8 oz. low fat cream cheese
1 Can of crabmeat
1/2 tsp. horse radish
Lemon juice

Instructions:
Mix cream cheese with crabmeat. Then add horse radish and lemon juice. Bake at
425 degrees for 25 min.

Crab Bites
By Chef Corin Szostek

Ingredients:
1 stick vegetable oil spread or margarine
1 jar light cheese spread
1/2 tsp. low fat mayonnaise
Dash of onion salt
1/2 tsp. garlic powder
1 Can crabmeat
8 Whole Wheat English Muffins

Instructions:
Let margarine and cheese soften to room temperature. Mix together with mayo, garlic and onion salt. Add crabmeat. Spread on English muffins. Put in freezer for 10 minutes. Then cut into quarters. Keep frozen until ready to use. Then place on cookie sheet and broil until bubbly crisp.

Triscuit Pizzas
By Michael J. Schiemer

Ingredients:
12 Low-Fat Triscuit Crackers
4-6 TBSP Tomato Sauce
2 Cups Fat Free Cheese
1-2 TBSP Italian Seasoning Powder

Instructions:
Place 12 Low-Fat Triscuit Crackers on a toaster oven pan. Add tomato sauce and fat free cheese to each one. Toast until cheese melted. Add Italian seasoning powder after they have been removed from the toaster oven. Can also be done on whole wheat English muffins.

Protein Smoothies
(Blender Required)

Chocolate Peanut Butter Cup
By Michael J. Schiemer

Ingredients:
6 Oz. Skim Milk
1 – 1.5 scoops of chocolate whey protein
2 Tbsp Natural Peanut Butter
Ice
1 Tbsp Cocoa Powder
1 Tbsp Chocolate Syrup (Sugar Free for weight loss)
1 TSP Splenda (optional)

Instructions:
Mix all ingredients together in blender making sure no peanut butter gets stuck on the sides. Feel free to add or subtract ice and skim milk for your preferred thickness. Serve as a breakfast or post-workout shake or just a healthy and filling snack.

The Cinnamon Bun
By Michael J. Schiemer

Ingredients:
10 oz. Skim Milk
1 – 1.5 scoops of vanilla whey protein
1 TBSP Cinnamon
4 oz yogurt
Ice

Instructions:
Mix all ingredients together in blender. Feel free to add or subtract ice, yogurt, and skim milk for preferred thickness.

Mocha Mania
By Michael J. Schiemer

Ingredients:
6 Oz. Skim Milk
1-1.5 Scoops chocolate whey protein
1 TBSP Cocoa Powder
2 TBSP mocha powder or instant coffee
Ice

Instructions:
Mix all ingredients together in blender for about 30-45 seconds. Feel free to add or subtract ice and skim milk for your preferred thickness. Serve as a breakfast or post-workout shake or just a healthy and filling snack. For even more of a coffee or mocha taste, switch out the chocolate whey protein for mocha or coffee flavored whey protein.

The Schiemer Shake (Lean Formula)
By Michael J. Schiemer

Ingredients:
12 oz Skim Milk
1 Scoop Dymatize Fudge Brownie Protein Powder
1 TBSP Natural Peanut Butter (optional)
2 TBSP Sugar Free Chocolate Syrup (optional)
Ice

Instructions:
Mix all ingredients together in blender for about 30-45 seconds. Feel free to add or subtract ice and skim milk for your preferred thickness. Serve as a breakfast or post-workout shake or just a healthy and filling snack.

The Schiemer Shake (Lean Formula) Lactose Intolerant
By Michael J. Schiemer

Ingredients:
12 oz Lactaid Milk
1 Scoop Chocolate Soy Protein Powder
1 TBSP Natural Peanut Butter (optional)
2 TBSP Sugar Free Chocolate Syrup (optional)
Ice

Instructions:
Mix all ingredients together in blender for about 30-45 seconds. Feel free to add or subtract ice and Lactaid milk for your preferred thickness. Serve as a breakfast or post-workout shake or just a healthy and filling snack.

The Schiemer Shake (Lean Formula) Vegan
By Michael J. Schiemer

Ingredients:
12 oz Soy Milk
1 Scoop Chocolate Soy Protein Powder
1 TBSP Natural Peanut Butter (optional)
2 TBSP Sugar Free Chocolate Syrup (optional)
Ice

Instructions:
Mix all ingredients together in blender for about 30-45 seconds. Feel free to add or subtract ice and soy milk for your preferred thickness. Serve as a breakfast or post-workout shake or just a healthy and filling snack.

The Schiemer Shake (Bulk-Up)
By Michael J. Schiemer

Ingredients:
12 oz Skim Milk
1.5 Scoops Dymatize Fudge Brownie Protein Powder
2 TBSP Natural Peanut Butter
2 TBSP Chocolate Syrup
1 TSP (5 grams) creatine monohydrate powder
Ice

Instructions:
Mix all ingredients together in blender for about 30-45 seconds. Feel free to add or subtract ice and skim milk for your preferred thickness. Serve as a breakfast or post-workout shake or just a healthy and filling snack if you are looking to put on muscle size and strength.

The Schiemer Fruit Shake (Bulk-Up)
By Michael J. Schiemer

Ingredients:
4 oz Yogurt
8 oz Cranberry Juice
1.5 Scoops Vanilla Protein Powder
1/2 Cup Raspberries
½ Cup Strawberries
1 Scoop Body Fortress Advanced Creatine Powder
Ice

Instructions:
Mix all ingredients together in blender for about 30-45 seconds. Drink immediately. Feel free to add or subtract ice, fruit, and fruit juice for your preferred thickness. Serve as a breakfast or post-workout shake or just a healthy and filling snack if you are looking to put on muscle size and strength.

The Schiemer Shake (Bulk-Up)
Lactose Intolerant
By Michael J. Schiemer

Ingredients:
12 oz Lactaid Milk
1.5 Scoops Chocolate Soy Protein Powder
2 TBSP Natural Peanut Butter
2 TBSP Chocolate Syrup
1 TSP (5 grams) creatine monohydrate powder
Ice

Instructions:
Mix all ingredients together in blender for about 30-45 seconds. Drink immediately. Feel free to add or subtract ice and Lactaid milk for your preferred thickness. Serve as a breakfast or post-workout shake or just a healthy and filling snack if you are looking to put on muscle size and strength.

The Schiemer Shake (Bulk-Up) Vegan
By Michael J. Schiemer

Ingredients:
12 oz Soy Milk
1.5 Scoops Chocolate Soy Protein
2 TBSP Natural Peanut Butter
2 TBSP Chocolate Syrup
1 TSP (5 grams) creatine monohydrate powder
Ice

Instructions:
Mix all ingredients together in blender for about 30-45 seconds. Feel free to add or subtract ice and soy milk for your preferred thickness. Serve as a breakfast or post-workout shake or just a healthy and filling snack if you are looking to put on muscle size and strength.

Fruity Tuity
By Michael J. Schiemer

Ingredients:
2/3 Cup Apple Juice (100% juice, not from concentrate)
2/3 Cup Cranberry Juice (100% juice, not from concentrate)
1.5 scoops vanilla or unflavored whey protein powder
1 Cup Raspberries
Ice

Instructions:
Mix all ingredients together in blender for about 30-45 seconds. Feel free to add or subtract ice and fruit for your preferred thickness. Serve as a breakfast or post-workout shake or just a healthy and filling snack. Do not consume at night unless it is post-workout due to its high sugar content.

Strawberry Shortcake Shake
By Michael J. Schiemer

Ingredients:
1 Cup Skim Milk
2 oz Fat Free Yogurt
1 scoops vanilla whey protein powder
1/2 Cup Strawberries
1 tsp cinnamon
1 tsp nutmeg
Ice

Instructions:
Mix all ingredients together in blender for about 30-45 seconds. Feel free to add or subtract ice and fruit for your preferred thickness. Serve as a breakfast or post-workout shake or just a healthy and filling snack.

Strawberry Fields Forever
By Michael J. Schiemer

Ingredients:
8 oz skim milk
4 oz nonfat yogurt
1 scoops vanilla whey protein powder
1 Cup strawberries
Ice

Instructions:
Mix all ingredients together in blender for about 30-45 seconds. Feel free to add or subtract ice and fruit for your preferred thickness. Serve as a breakfast or post-workout shake or just a healthy and filling snack.

Razzleberry Razz
By Michael J. Schiemer

Ingredients:
½ Cup Skim Milk
2 oz nonfat yogurt
1 scoop vanilla whey protein powder
1 Cup Raspberries
Ice

Instructions:
Mix all ingredients together in blender for about 30-45 seconds. Feel free to add or subtract ice and fruit for your preferred thickness. Serve as a breakfast or post-workout shake or just a healthy and filling snack.

Razzleberry Razz (Vegan)
By Michael J. Schiemer

Ingredients:
½ Cup Soy Milk
2 oz Soy Yogurt
1 scoop vanilla soy protein powder
1 Cup Raspberries
Ice

Instructions:
Mix all ingredients together in blender for about 30-45 seconds. Feel free to add or subtract ice and fruit for your preferred thickness. Serve as a breakfast or post-workout shake or just a healthy and filling snack.

Chocolate Banana Blast
By Michael J. Schiemer

Ingredients:
1 Banana
1 Scoop Chocolate Protein Powder
1 Cup Skim or Soy Milk
1 TBSP Chocolate Syrup (sugar free for weight loss)
Ice

Instructions:
Mix all ingredients together in blender for about 30-45 seconds. Feel free to add or subtract ice and milk for your preferred thickness. Serve as a breakfast or post-workout shake or just a healthy and filling snack.

Chocolate Peanut Butter Banana Bonanza
By Michael J. Schiemer

Ingredients:
1 Banana
1 Scoop Chocolate Protein Powder
1-2 TBSP Natural Peanut Butter
10 oz Skim or Soy Milk
1 TBSP Chocolate Syrup (sugar free for weight loss)
Ice

Instructions:
Mix all ingredients together in blender for about 30-45 seconds. Feel free to add or subtract ice and milk for your preferred thickness. Serve as a breakfast or post-workout shake or just a healthy and filling snack

Chocolate Minty Mayhem
By Michael J. Schiemer

Ingredients:
1 Scoop Chocolate Mint Protein Powder
Mint Leaves (optional)
1 TBSP Cocoa Powder
10 oz Skim or Soy Milk
1 TBSP Chocolate Syrup (sugar free for weight loss)
Ice

Instructions:
Mix all ingredients together in blender for about 30-45 seconds. Feel free to add or subtract ice and milk for your preferred thickness. Serve as a breakfast or post-workout shake or just a healthy and filling snack.

Banana Soy Smoothie (Vegan)
By Lori Cushner

Ingredients:
10 oz Soy Milk or Vanilla Soy Milk
1 Banana or Frozen Banana Slices
Nuts (optional)
Shredded Coconut (optional)
Ice

Instructions:
Mix all ingredients together in blender for about 30-45 seconds. Feel free to add or subtract ice and fruit for your preferred thickness. Serve as a breakfast or post-workout shake or just a healthy and filling snack.

Banana Smoothie (Lactose Intolerant)
By Lori Cushner and Michael J. Schiemer

Ingredients:
12 oz Lactaid Milk
½ Scoop Vanilla Soy Protein Powder
1 Banana or Frozen Banana Slices
Nuts (optional)
Shredded Coconut (optional)
Ice

Instructions:
Mix all ingredients together in blender for about 30-45 seconds. Feel free to add or subtract ice and fruit for your preferred thickness. Serve as a breakfast or post-workout shake or just a healthy and filling snack.

Ultimate Power Fruit Smoothie
By Michael J. Schiemer

Ingredients:
12-16 oz water
1 EmergenC raspberry packet
1 Energy Rush berry packet
1 Scoop Body Fortress Advanced Creatine powder
Ice

Instructions:
Mix all ingredients together in blender. After initial fizzing subsides, drink quickly for a huge rush of sugar, caffeine, B-vitamins, and creatine. Best when waking up or 30 minutes pre-workout, only if you are trying to put on weight.

The Blueberry Muffin
By Michael J. Schiemer

Ingredients:
12 oz Skim Milk
1.5 Scoop Vanilla or Blueberry Muffin Protein Powder
2/3 Cup Blueberries
2 oz Yogurt
Ice

Instructions:
Mix all ingredients together in blender for about 30-45 seconds. Feel free to add or subtract ice, yogurt, milk, or fruit for your preferred thickness. Serve as a breakfast, post-workout shake, or just a healthy and filling snack.

Home-Made Whey Protein
By Nicholas Sullivan

Ingredients:
1 quart or liter of milk
2 TBSP Vinegar or lemon juice
Any flavoring or spices you want
(cinnamon, nutmeg, cocoa, honey, vanilla)

Cooking Utensils:
Strainer
Saucepan
Paper Towels or Cheese Cloth

Instructions:
Get your milk and start to boil it on a medium to low heat. Keep a close eye on it because you don't want it to get too hot. When you start to see bubbling around the rim of the sauce pan, add the vinegar or lemon juice and stir. The mixture should separate pretty quickly into curds and whey. If it doesn't just add a little more vinegar or lemon juice until it does. The curds are the solid parts and the whey is the liquid. Get a strainer (cover it in paper towels or cheese cloth if you want to keep the curds and make it into cheese). Separate the curds from the whey. Let the whey cool down in the fridge for a while and then add any ingredients. Some suggestions for flavoring: Nutmeg, cinnamon, honey, chocolate, vanilla. The taste might be different for some people if it is, just dilute it with something else like water, or juice. There are other ways of drying it as well such as taking the liquid and leaving it uncovered over a low heat on the stove, this should allow excess water to evaporate off and leave a more concentrated solution. Place remaining solid in a grinder if you need to refine it. This is very similar to the stuff you'll buy in the store except it's not dehydrated and probably won't have any additional additives.

<u>Desserts</u>

Oatmeal Cookies:
By Chef Corin Szostek

Makes: About 50 Cookies

Ingredients:
2 1/2 chips uncooked oats
1 1/2 cups whole wheat flour
1/2 teaspoon cinnamon
1/2 teaspoon baking soda
1/4 teaspoon salt(optional)
1 cup honey or maple syrup (sugar free if you want)
3/4 cup softened margarine or butter
1/2 teaspoon vanilla extract
1 egg
1/2 cup chopped nuts (optional)
1/2 cup raisins (optional)

Instructions:
Heat oven to 375 degrees F. lightly coat cookie sheet with vegetable oil or non-stick cooking spray. Combine dry ingredients, mix well. Mix honey, margarine and vanilla until smooth. Add egg. Blend dry ingredients, mixing thoroughly. Stir in raisins, nuts if you desire. Place rounded spoonfuls of blended ingredients onto cookie sheet. Bake for approximately 10 minutes. Cool and enjoy!

Raisin Bran Cookies
By Chef Corin Szostek

Makes: About 48 Cookies

Ingredients:
1 cup raisins
1/2 cup butter or margarine
1 cup Splenda brown Sugar mix
1 egg
1/2 cup fat free skim milk
2 cups oat bran
2 cups whole wheat flour
1 tablespoon baking powder
1/4 teaspoon salt

Instructions:
Preheat the oven to 275 degrees F. In a mixing bowl, cream the butter with the brown sugar. Beat in the eggs and the milk. In another bowl, combine the bran, flour, baking powder and salt. Work the wet ingredients together with the fry to form a stiff batter. Then work in the raisins. Scoop out the cookie dough onto lightly butter or sprayed with non stick cooking spray like Pam cookie sheets and press down lightly with a wet fork. Bake for 10 minutes, until firm and lightly browned.

Chocolate-Filled Raspberries
By Heather Mayer and Sarah Klein

Ingredients:
One carton of raspberries, the bigger the holes the better
Chocolate or dark chocolate morsels or pieces of a bar

Directions:
The time to prepare treat is about 15-20 minutes. Melt chocolate - this can be done on a double boiler or in the microwave. If done in the microwave, heat for periods of 10-15 seconds and stir so the chocolate doesn't burn. Fill a baggie/frosting bag with melted chocolate. Slowly squeeze a little bit of chocolate into the hole of each raspberry - don't overflow too much. Refrigerate until the chocolate is hard. Try using dark chocolate for extra antioxidant content and reduced added sugar.

Perfect Protein Bars
By Chef Corin Szostek

Ingredients:
2 cups cooking oats
1/2 cup natural peanut butter
4 scoops of chocolate protein powder
1 Tsp ground flaxseed
1/2 cup water

Instructions:
Mix all ingredients together in a bowl until thoroughly combined. Use a square 8"x 8" baking pan with wax paper. Press dough into bottom of pan. Freeze for 30 minutes. Cut into bars. Store in refrigerator.

Approximate Nutrition Content: (Per Serving), Calories: 230, fats: 10 g, Sat fat: 2 g, sodium: 20 mg, carbs: 21 g, fiber: 4 g, sugars: 3 g, protein: 15 g

Multi-Grain Cookies
By Chef Corin Szostek

Makes: About 50 Cookies

Ingredients:
3 cups uncooked Whole Grain or Multigrain Cereal
1 1/2 cups whole wheat flour
1/2 teaspoon cinnamon
1/2 teaspoon baking soda
1/4 teaspoon salt (Optional)
1 cup honey or maple syrup (sugar free if desired)
3/4 cup butter or margarine
1/2 teaspoon vanilla extract
1 Egg
1/2 cup nuts (Optional)
1/2 cup Raisins (Optional)

Instructions:
Heat oven to 375 degrees F. Lightly coat cookie sheet with vegetable oil or non stick fat free cooking spray. Combine dry ingredients, mix well. Mix honey, and vanilla until smooth. Add egg. Blend dry ingredients, mixing thoroughly. Stir in (optional) raisins, and or nuts. Place rounded spoonfuls of blended ingredients onto cookie sheet. Bake approximately 10 minutes. Cool and enjoy.

Pumpkin-Raisin Spice Bread
By Chef Corin Szostek

Ingredients:
3/4 cup canned pumpkin, unsweetened
1/2 cup evaporated cane juice
1 cup molasses
4 tablespoons canola oil
3/4 cup buttermilk or fat free milk
1 tablespoon vanilla extract
4 large egg whites
2 cups rolled oats or cooking oats
1 1/2 cups whole wheat flour
1 tablespoon baking powder
12 teaspoon nutmeg
1/2 teaspoon cinnamon
1/8 teaspoon salt (optional)
1/2 cup raisins and/or nuts of your choice (optional)

Instructions:
Preheat oven to 350 degrees f. Spray a large loaf pan with non stick cooking spray. Mix the first seven ingredients together. Add in 1 1/2 cups oats, and the other remaining ingredients; blend until just mixed. Pour dough evenly into prepared pan, filling it only about 3/4 full. Sprinkle top with remaining cup of oats. Bake for 30-45 minutes, or until top is slightly soft to touch, but not wet. Allow to cool before removing from pan.

Apple Cake
By Chef Corin Szostek

Ingredients:
4 c. diced apples
3 c. flour
1 tsp. salt
2. c sugar
2 tsp. cinnamon
1 tsp. baking powder
1. c. olive oil
2 beaten eggs
1/2 c. chopped walnuts (optional)

Instructions:
Put all but apples into a bowl and mix until moistened. Add apples. Bake at 350 degrees for 1 hour and 15 minutes. Bundt pan works well. Sprinkle with confectioner's sugar after cake cooled.

Healthier Hot Chocolate
By Michael J. Schiemer

Makes: 1 Large Cup

Ingredients:
10 oz. Skim Milk
1 Tbsp Cocoa Powder
1 Tbsp Sugar Free Chocolate Syrup
1 Drop Vanilla Extract (optional)
1 TSP Splenda (optional)

Instructions:
Heat or microwave a large coffee cup filled with skim milk. Add Cocoa powder and mix thoroughly. Add sugar free chocolate syrup, vanilla extract, and/or Splenda and mix thoroughly again.

Light and Sweet Chocolate Chai Tea Latte
By Michael J. Schiemer

Makes: 16 oz Cup

Ingredients:
12 oz. boiling water
2 Chai Tea Bags
1 Tbsp Cocoa Powder
4 oz Skim milk or vanilla soy milk
1 Drop Vanilla Extract (optional)
2 Splenda packets (optional)

Instructions:
Start with a 16 oz or larger cup with 12 oz of boiling water. Add the 2 chai tea bags and cocoa powder and let them sit for a minute. Then add the skim or soy milk, vanilla extract, and/or Splenda packets. Mix thoroughly and drink hot or save for later to drink with ice cubes.

VII

Frugalicious Meal Plans

All of the delicious frugal recipes and nutrition tips mean very little unless you can organize them all into convenient daily meal plans that work for you and your schedule. These meal plans are excellent ideas for you based on your estimated caloric intake mentioned earlier. What is even better is you can mix and match these foods, meals, or snacks to suit your schedule, food preferences, and budget. These don't have to be followed to the letter! Also, I normally do not recommend meal plans under 1,500 calories for anyone but sometimes there are people that could utilize these plans (an individual that is very petite, small, light, and/or sedentary) so they are included just in case down to 1,200 calories. On the flip side, there are also some people (young, athlete, bodybuilder, high activity level, and/or high metabolism) that are looking to put on muscle that may need more than 3,500 calories. The meal plans included should cover the caloric needs of about 99% of the people out there. The elite bodybuilders and athletes will have to modify the meal plans themselves to include more meals and calories. The Frugal Recipes from the last chapter are also not included in most of these meal plans so feel free to substitute in the ones you like for some of the generic meal options. Enjoy the meal plans and get your daily and weekly nutrition organized!

Get Lean Meal Plan (1,200 Calories)

Breakfast:
- -1 Bowl of Total Cereal with skim milk
- -1 8 oz Cup Skim Milk
- -Cup Black Coffee
- - Multivitamin and 2 Flaxseed Oil Capsules

Snack #1:
- -Handful of blueberries
- -5 Low Fat Wheat Thin Crackers

Lunch:
- -Half turkey sandwich on whole wheat bread
- -Green Tea
- -Apple

Snack #2:
- -Celery and carrot sticks
- -5 Almonds

Dinner:
- -3 oz baked, broiled, or grilled Chicken Breast, skinless
- -1 cup edamame
- -1 Cup Green Beans
- -Chamomile Tea

Water and/or Decaffeinated Tea Throughout The Day!

Get Lean Meal Plan (1,300 Calories)

Breakfast: -1 Cup of Cooked Oatmeal with Splenda
Brown Sugar
-1 8 oz Cup Skim Milk
-1 Cup Orange Juice
-Cup Coffee with Skim Milk and Splenda
- Multivitamin and 2 Flaxseed Oil Capsules

Snack #1:   -Fat Free Yogurt

Lunch: -2 oz Turkey Breast, Spicy Mustard, Lettuce,
on Whole Grain Bread
-Green Tea
-Celery sticks

Snack #2:   -1 Cup Blueberries

Dinner: -3 oz baked, broiled, or grilled Chicken
Breast, skinless
-Steamed Broccoli
-Decaf Green Tea

Snack #3:   -Half a glass (4 oz) of Skim Milk

Water and/or Decaffeinated Tea Throughout The Day!

Get Lean Meal Plan (1,400 Calories)

Breakfast: -1 Cup of Cooked Oatmeal with Banana
               Slices
               -1 8 oz Cup Skim Milk
               -1 Cup Orange Juice
               -Cup Coffee with Skim Milk and Splenda
               (optional)
               - Multivitamin and 2 Flaxseed Oil Capsules

Snack #1:   -Fat Free Cottage Cheese

Lunch: -2 oz Turkey Breast, Spicy Mustard, Lettuce,
               on Whole Grain Bread
               -5 Low Fat Wheat Thin Crackers
               -Green Tea
               -Cup of Carrots

Snack #2:   -1 Small box of raisins

Dinner: -3 oz baked, broiled, or grilled Chicken
               Breast, skinless
               -1 Spinach with garlic and oil
               -1 Cup Green Beans
               -Decaf Green Tea

Snack #3:   -Half a glass (4 oz) of Skim Milk

Water and/or Decaffeinated Tea Throughout The Day!

Get Lean Meal Plan (1,500 Calories)

Breakfast: -1 Cup of Cooked Oatmeal with Splenda
Brown Sugar
-1 8 oz Cup Skim Milk
-1 Cup Orange Juice
-Cup Coffee with Skim Milk and Splenda
- Multivitamin and 2 Flaxseed Oil Capsules

Snack #1:   -Fat Free Yogurt

Lunch: -Grilled Chicken and Lettuce in a whole
wheat pita wrap, light dressing
-Green Tea
-Cup of Carrots

Snack #2:   -1 Cup Blueberries

Dinner: -3 oz baked, broiled, or grilled Chicken
Breast, skinless
-1 Medium Sweet Potato
-1 Cup Green Beans
-Decaf Green Tea

Snack #3:   -3 Cups of Light or Low-Fat Popcorn

Water and/or Decaffeinated Tea Throughout The Day!

Get Lean Meal Plan (1,600 Calories)

Breakfast: -2 Slices Whole Wheat Toast with margarine
               -1 Cup Green Tea
               -1 Cup Skim Milk
               - Multivitamin and 2 Flaxseed Oil Capsules

Snack #1:   -1 whole wheat pita with tabouli

Lunch: -Light Salad
               -1 Whole Grain Roll,
               -1 Cup Black Tea

Snack #2:   -1 Cup Strawberries

Dinner: -3 oz baked, broiled, or grilled Chicken
               Breast, skinless
               -1 Cup Brown Rice
               -Carrots
               -Decaf Green Tea

Snack #3:   -Scoop of casein protein in water

Water and/or Decaffeinated Tea Throughout The Day!

Get Lean Meal Plan (1,700 Calories)

Breakfast: -2 Whole Grain Pancakes with Blueberries
and Sugar Free Maple Syrup
-1 Cup Green Tea
-1 Cup Skim Milk
- Multivitamin and 2 Flaxseed Oil Capsules

Snack #1:   -1 Tbsp Hummus with Celery Sticks

Lunch: -Salad with lettuce, carrots, green peppers,
cabbage, grilled chicken, parmesan cheese,
and light or self-made dressing
-1 Whole Grain Roll,
-1 Cup Black Tea

Snack #2:   -1 Peach

Dinner: -3 oz baked, broiled, or grilled Chicken
Breast, skinless
-1 Cup Brown Rice
-Carrots
-Decaf Green Tea

Snack #3:   -1 Low Fat Yogurt with nuts

Water and/or Decaffeinated Tea Throughout The Day!

Get Lean Meal Plan (1,800 Calories)

Breakfast: -1 Cup of Cooked Oatmeal with Whey
              Protein Powder and Splenda
              -1 8 oz Cup Skim Milk
              -1 Cup Orange Juice
              -Cup Coffee with Skim Milk and Splenda
              - Multivitamin and 2 Flaxseed Oil Capsules

Snack #1:   -Banana with Natural Peanut Butter

Lunch: -3 oz Turkey Breast, Spicy Mustard, Lettuce,
              Tomato on Whole Grain Bread
              -Green Tea
              -Grapefruit

Snack #2:   -1 Cup Blueberries

Dinner: -Chicken Burger with low fat cheese, BBQ
              sauce, on whole grain bun
              -8 oz Glass of Skim Milk
              -Decaf Green Tea

Snack #3:   -1 Scoop Whey Protein in water

Water and/or Decaffeinated Tea Throughout The Day!

Get Lean Meal Plan (1,900 Calories)

Breakfast: -3 Scrambled Eggs
-2 Pieces of Multigrain or Wheat Toast w/ margarine
-Apple, Orange, or Banana
-Cup Coffee with Skim Milk and Splenda
- Multivitamin and 2 Flaxseed Oil Capsules

Snack #1:   -Fat Free Yogurt with nuts or ground flax seed added
-Handful of Roasted Peanuts

Lunch: -Spinach Salad, Grilled Chicken, Parmesan Cheese, Garlic, Olive Oil
-Green Tea
-Bag of Baked Lays

Snack #2:   -Half Can of Tuna
-Handful of Kashi Heart to Heart Toasted Honey Cereal

Dinner: -Serving of Whole Wheat Pasta, Tomato Sauce, Garlic and/or Parmesan Cheese, spices.
-Water or Decaf Tea
-Grilled Chicken or Lean Beef

Snack #3:   -Cup of Oatmeal w/skim milk, almonds, cinnamon, and Splenda

Water and/or Decaffeinated Tea Throughout The Day!

Get Lean Meal Plan (2,000 Calories)

Breakfast: -Cup of Oatmeal w/Skim Milk
                  -Glass of Orange Juice
                  - Skim Milk and Whey Protein Powder
Scoop
                  -Multivitamin and 2 Flaxseed Oil Capsules

Snack #1:   -Whey Protein Drink
                  -Piece of Fruit

Lunch: -2-3 Slices Chicken Breast cold cuts, Piece of
                  Cheese, Tomato Slice, Lettuce, 1 tsp Smart
                  Balance Mayo on Wheat/Multigrain Bread
                  -Cup of Green Tea
                  -10 Low Fat Triscuit Crackers

Snack #2:   -Glass of skim milk
                  -Kashi Crunchy Granola Bar

Dinner: -Whole Wheat Pasta w/Tomato Sauce,
                  Garlic, and Parmesan Cheese
                  -1 Cup Steamed Broccoli
                  -Water or Decaf Tea

Snack #3:   - 8 oz Cup of Skim Milk

Water and/or Decaffeinated Tea Throughout The Day!

Get Lean Meal Plan (2,100 Calories)

Breakfast: -Cup of Kashi Heart to Heart Honey Toasted Cereal w/ skim milk & strawberries
-Skim Milk Plus Scoop of protein powder
-Multivitamin and 2 Flaxseed Oil Capsules
-Black Tea

Snack #1:   -PowerBar Triple Threat Peanut Butter Chocolate Crisp

Lunch: -Tuna Melt on Rye Toast, Low-fat Cheese, No Mayo
-Diet Soda or Tea
-Handful of Sun Chips

Snack #2:   -Serving of Beef Jerky
-10 Kashi Whole Grain Crackers
-Water

Dinner: -Salmon or Chicken Stir Fry with Brown Rice, Veggies, soy sauce, garlic
-Decaf Tea or water

Snack #3:   -Glass of skim milk with protein powder scoop

Water and/or Decaffeinated Tea Throughout The Day!

Get Lean Meal Plan (2,200 Calories)

Breakfast: -Cup of Kashi Heart to Heart Blueberry
Cluster Cereal w/ skim milk
-Skim Milk Plus Scoop of protein powder
-Scoop of natural peanut butter
-Multivitamin and 2 Flaxseed Oil Capsules
-Tea with lemon

Snack #1:   -South Beach Diet High Protein Chocolate
Bar

Lunch: -Tuna Melt on Rye Toast, Low-fat Cheese,
No Mayo
-Diet Soda or Tea
-Handful of Sun Chips

Snack #2:   -Serving of Beef Jerky
-10 Wheat Thins
-Water

Dinner: -Salmon or Chicken Stir Fry with Brown
Rice, Veggies, soy sauce, garlic
-Decaf Tea or water

Snack #3:   -Glass of skim milk with protein powder
scoop

Water and/or Decaffeinated Tea Throughout The Day!

Get Lean Meal Plan (2,300 Calories)

Breakfast:
-Cup of Total Raisin Bran Cereal w/ skim milk
-Skim Milk Plus Scoop of protein powder
-Scoop of natural peanut butter
-Multivitamin and 2 Flaxseed Oil Capsules
-Orange Pekoe Tea

Snack #1:
-Low Fat Yogurt
-Orange

Lunch:
-Chicken Caesar Salad with light dressing and low fat cheese
-Diet Soda or coffee
-Handful of Sun Chips

Snack #2:
-Serving of Fat Free Cottage Cheese
-10 Kashi Whole Grain Crackers
-Water

Dinner:
-Salmon or Chicken Stir Fry with Brown Rice, Veggies, soy sauce, garlic
-Whole Grain Roll with margarine/vegetable oil buttery spread

Snack #3:
-8 oz Glass of skim milk with protein powder scoop

Water and/or Decaffeinated Tea Throughout The Day!

Get Lean Meal Plan (2,400 Calories)

Breakfast: -Bowl of oatmeal with pecans, blueberries,
              and flaxseed or wheat germ
              -Skim Milk Plus Scoop of protein powder
              -Scoop of natural peanut butter
              -Multivitamin and 2 Flaxseed Oil Capsules
              -White Tea

Snack #1:   -Low Fat Yogurt
              -Orange

Lunch: -1 Slice Veggie Pizza on wheat or whole
              grain crust
              -Crystal Light in water
              -Bag of Baked Lays Potato Chips

Snack #2:   -Serving of Fat Free Cottage Cheese
              -Handful of Total cereal

Dinner: -Chicken Caesar Salad, light dressing
              -Whole Grain Roll with margarine
              -Decaf Tea or water

Snack #3:   -8 oz Glass of skim milk with protein powder
              scoop

Water and/or Decaffeinated Tea Throughout The Day!

Get Lean Meal Plan (2,500 Calories)

Breakfast: -Veggie Omelette
              -Multivitamin and 2 Flaxseed Oil Capsules
              -Coffee with skim milk and Splenda
              (optional)

Snack #1:   -Hummus with 2 whole grain pitas

Lunch: -Grilled Chicken and Veggie wrap with
              whole wheat pita
              -Crystal Light in water
              -Bag of Baked Lays Potato Chips

Snack #2:   -Scoop of Whey protein and water

Dinner: -Turkey breast
              -Sweet Potato
              -Spinach Salad with light dressing and cheese
              -Whole Grain Roll with margarine
              -Decaf Tea or water

Snack #3:   -8 oz Glass of skim milk with protein powder
              scoop

Water and/or Decaffeinated Tea Throughout The Day!

Get Big Meal Plan (3,000 Calories)

Breakfast: -1/2 Scoop of Body Fortress Advanced Creatine in 10 oz water
- Skim Milk and Scoop of Protein Powder
-4 Slices of Multigrain Toast with margarine
-Multivitamin and 2 Flaxseed Oil Capsules

Snack #1: -Tbsp of Natural Peanut Butter
-Can of Tuna
-Handful of Kashi Heart To Heart Toasted Honey cereal

Lunch: -3 Slices Chicken Breast, 2 Slices Low-Fat Cheese, 2 Tomato Slices, Lettuce, 1 tsp Smart Balance Mayo on Wheat/Multigrain Bread
-Cup of Green Tea
-8 oz of Skim Milk
-10-15 Low Fat Triscuit Crackers

Snack #2: -12 oz Skim Milk with scoop Protein Powder
-Kashi Crunchy Granola Bar

Dinner: -3 Cups Whole Wheat Pasta w/Tomato Sauce, Garlic, and Parmesan Cheese
-1 Cup Steamed Broccoli
-Decaf Tea

Snack #3: -12 oz Skim Milk with scoop of Dymatize 12 Hour Elite Protein powder
-Multivitamin and 2 Flaxseed Oil Capsules

Water and/or Decaffeinated Tea Throughout The Day!

Get Big Meal Plan (3,100 Calories)

Breakfast: (800 cal)	-Multivitamin and 2 Flaxseed Oil Capsules -12 oz Glass of Orange Juice -EmergenC + Energy Rush Packet in water - Skim Milk and Scoop of Protein Powder -2 bowls Kashi Cereal with Skim Milk
Snack #1:	-2 Scoops of Chocolate Peanut Butter Crisp -Handful of Kashi Cereal
Lunch:	-Subway Grilled Chicken Footlong with Cheese on Multigrain Bread -Energy Rush + EmergenC packets in water -Bag of Sunchips
Snack #2:	-12 oz Skim Milk with scoop of Dymatize 12 Hour Elite Protein powder -Bag of Low-Fat microwaved popcorn
Dinner:	-Lean Beef Burger with BBQ Sauce, Low-Fat Cheese, Lettuce, Tomato -1 Cup Steamed Broccoli -8 oz Glass of Skim Milk -Decaf Tea
Snack #3:	-12 oz Skim Milk with scoop of Dymatize 12 Hour Elite Protein powder -Handful of Total cereal -Multivitamin and 2 Flaxseed Oil Capsules

Water and/or Decaffeinated Tea Throughout The Day!

Get Big Meal Plan (3,200 Calories)

Breakfast: -Multivitamin and 2 Flaxseed Oil Capsules
                  -Scoop of Body Fortress Advanced Creatine
                  in Water
                  -EmergenC + Energy Rush Packet in water
                  -Scoop of natural peanut butter
                  - Skim Milk and Scoop of Protein Powder
                  -2 bowls Kashi Cereal with Skim Milk

Snack #1:   -2 Scoops of Chocolate Peanut Butter Crisp
                  -Handful of Total cereal
                  -Orange

Lunch: -Tuna Melt
                  -Energy Rush and EmergenC packets in 12
                  oz water
                  -Bag of Sunchips
                  -Banana

Snack #2:   -12 oz Skim Milk with scoop of Protein
                  Powder
                  -Bag of Low-Fat microwaved popcorn

Dinner: -Lean Chicken Burger with BBQ Sauce,
                  Low-Fat Cheese, Lettuce, Tomato
                  -2 Cup Steamed Broccoli
                  -8 oz Glass of Skim Milk

Snack #3:   -12 oz Skim Milk with scoop of Protein
                  Powder
                  -Bowl of Kashi cereal with nuts
                  -Multivitamin and 2 Flaxseed Oil Capsules

Water and/or Decaffeinated Tea Throughout The Day!

Get Big Meal Plan (3,300 Calories)

Breakfast: -Multivitamin and 2 Flaxseed Oil Capsules
-Scoop of Body Fortress Advanced Creatine in Water
-EmergenC and Energy Rush Packet in water
-Scoop of natural peanut butter
- Skim Milk and Scoop Protein powder
-2 bowls Kashi with 1/2 cup Skim Milk and fruit

Snack #1:   -2 Scoops of Chocolate Peanut Butter Crisp
-Handful of Total cereal
-Orange

Lunch: -Subway Grilled Chicken Footlong with Cheese, Lettuce, Tomatoes, Peppers, and Onions on Multigrain Bread
-Energy Rush and EmergenC packets in 12 oz water
-Bag of Sunchips
-Banana

Snack #2:   -12 oz Skim Milk with scoop Protein Powder
-Bag of Low-Fat microwaved popcorn

Dinner: -Grilled Chicken Sandwich
-Sweet Potato
-2 Cup Steamed Broccoli
-8 oz Glass of Skim Milk

Snack #3:   -12 oz Skim Milk with scoop Protein Powder
-Bowl of Kashi cereal with fruit and nuts
-Multivitamin and 2 Flaxseed Oil Capsules

Water and/or Decaffeinated Tea Throughout The Day!

Get Big Meal Plan (3,400 Calories)

Breakfast: -Multivitamin and 2 Flaxseed Oil Capsules
               -Scoop of Body Fortress Advanced Creatine
               in Water
               -EmergenC and Energy Rush Packet in water
               -Scoop of natural peanut butter
               - Skim Milk and Scoop of Protein Powder
               -2 bowls Kashi Cereal with 1/2 cup Skim
               Milk and Fruit

Snack #1:   -2 Scoops of Chocolate Peanut Butter Crisp
               -Handful of Total cereal
               -Orange

Lunch: -Subway Meatball Sub Foot-Long
               -Energy Rush and EmergenC packets in
               water
               -Bag of Sunchips
               -Banana

Snack #2:   -12 oz Skim Milk with scoop of Protein
               Powder
               -Bag of Low-Fat microwaved popcorn

Dinner: -Whole Grain Chicken Quesadillas with salsa
               -2 Cup Steamed Broccoli
               -8 oz Glass of Skim Milk

Snack #3:   -12 oz Skim Milk with scoop of Protein
               Powder
               -Bowl of oatmeal with nuts, fruit, and flax
               -Multivitamin and 2 Flaxseed Oil Capsules

Water and/or Decaffeinated Tea Throughout The Day!

Get Big Meal Plan (3,500 Calories)

Breakfast:
- Multivitamin and 2 Flaxseed Oil Capsules
- Scoop of Body Fortress Advanced Creatine in Water
- EmergenC + Energy Rush Packet in water
- Scoop of natural peanut butter
- Skim Milk and Scoop Protein Powder
- 2 bowls oatmeal with 1/2 cup Skim Milk, nuts, and fruit

Snack #1:
- 2 Scoops of Chocolate Peanut Butter Crisp
- Handful of Total cereal
- Orange

Lunch:
- Bacon Lettuce Tomato Subway Footlong
- Energy Rush and EmergenC packets in 12 oz water
- Bag of Sunchips
- Banana

Snack #2:
- 12 oz Skim Milk with scoop of Protein Powder
- Bag of Low-Fat microwaved popcorn

Dinner:
- Grilled Chicken Stir-Fry
- 2 Whole Grain Rolls with margarine
- 8 oz Glass of Skim Milk

Snack #3:
- 12 oz Skim Milk with scoop of Protein Powder
- Bowl of Kashi Heart to Heart Toasted Honey cereal
- Multivitamin and 2 Flaxseed Oil Capsules

Water and/or Decaffeinated Tea Throughout The Day!

__Homeless Meal Plan (1,600 Calories)__

Breakfast: -1 Cup 100% Rolled Oats
     -8-12 oz whole milk
     -1 Scoop Peanut Butter
     -1 Multivitamin

Snack: # 1 -Apple, Orange, or Banana

Lunch: -1 Cup 100% Rolled Oats
     -1 Can of Tuna

Snack #2: -8-12 oz whole milk

Dinner: -1 Cup 100% Rolled Oats
     -8-12 oz whole milk
     -1 Scoop Peanut Butter
     -1 Multivitamin

Free water throughout the day!

VIII

Frugal Nutritional Supplements

Why Use Nutritional Supplements?

Reality:
You may have heard from your doctor or read in a magazine that you don't need any supplements in your diet to be healthy and at peak performance. These people always make the claim that "you should be getting all of your nutrients from a healthy and balanced diet" and that supplements are a waste of money. They are right in a way, ideally we should be getting all of the nutrients from a healthy and balanced diet. Does that ever actually happen? Almost never! Guess

what, a lot of these doctors, registered dietitians, and writers that claim you don't need nutritional supplements are overweight and unhealthy! It's time to stop living in an imaginary world where everyone carries around Tupperware containers filled with broccoli and chicken breasts everywhere they go. Here are just a few reasons why we need healthy nutritional supplements in our diet.

Most Of Us Eat Horribly:
We (hopefully) know that a healthy and balanced diet should consist of whole grains, lots of fruits and veggies, legumes, low-fat dairy, and lean meats. What does the average diet actually include? It ends up being more like a coffee and sugary cereal for breakfast, a fatty sandwich with a soda for lunch, and pizza for dinner. This leaves massive holes in the diet for proper protein, carbohydrate, and fat intake as well as vitamin and mineral deficiencies. What does that mean to you? It means that without the right amounts of these nutrients you will have reduced mental focus, increased fat storage, reduced recovery rates from exercise, poor physical performance, and less immunity to sickness. Even vegetarians (who claim they're healthier than the average omnivore) usually need to supplement with extra protein and a multivitamin/multimineral because they aren't taking enough in from their normal diet. Healthy supplements such as Whey Protein, Multivitamin/Multiminerals, Tea, and Omega-3 capsules can help fill in these inevitable nutritional gaps.

Optimal Performance:
Not all of us have the same nutritional needs. Our requirements are based largely on our genetics and activity levels, not everyone is going to fit in with the

Recommended Daily Allowance's minimal range of nutrient intakes. An athlete or very active person is going to require larger amounts of nutrients than a couch potato (Kraemer et al, 1998). It is common sense that somebody trying to put on muscle needs to increase their protein and calorie intake to provide the raw materials for building that muscle (Chandler et al, 1994). What is the easiest way to boost up that protein intake? A whey protein shake, of course. It is a lot easier and cheaper to take 10 seconds and mix up a shake than to cook up some eggs or chicken breasts and then clean up. Distance runners need much larger amounts of carbohydrates than the typical person because they use up huge amounts during a run for energy. Before, during, and after a race they can supplement their carbohydrate levels with quick and effective supplements such as sports drinks, or Gel packs. I'm pretty sure runners aren't going to carry around rice cakes and pasta during a marathon for mid-race carbohydrate replenishment, so once again supplements are convenient, practical, and effective.

My Top Frugal Supplements:

Green Tea

General Information: The benefits of green tea have been known for thousands of years. Green tea bags are considered food products while green tea with added herbs and green tea extract are considered dietary supplements. I would recommend at least 1-2 cups a day for increased metabolism and improved immune system. Green Tea Extract works similar to this but possibly to a lesser extent but it can be more convenient at times. (Don't drink later than mid-afternoon or it may disturb your sleeping habits, unless drinking Decaf Green Tea). Green Tea has a very high concentration of antioxidants which help to positively stimulate your immune system to fight off sickness and excessive free radicals. Green Tea also has a very high concentration of ECGC, as well as small-moderate amounts of caffeine, that significantly improve fat-burning. While Green Tea may not miraculously burn 10 lbs of fat overnight, it is an excellent addition to a fat loss diet and exercise regimen. Try substituting a cup or two of Green Tea instead of your coffee to improve overall health. Green tea extract is not as potent as the regular tea form so try to drink more instead. Bottoms up for better health!

Cost: A box of 20 tea bags will cost you around $4, you can usually get a much cheaper price if you buy store brand, unflavored, and/or in bulk. I've gotten 100 black tea or orange pekoe tea bags for $1 so there are definitely low enough prices out there for anyone's price range. Green tea is usually slightly more expensive but you can get about 100 green tea bags for no more than $2 or $3. Green tea extract capsules are usually about $10 for 100 capsules but price may vary greatly depending on brand and what store you buy them.

Risks/Side Effects: See "A Note On Caffeine" but green tea has significantly less caffeine than coffee or other caffeine supplements.

Multivitamin/Multimineral

General Information: Multivitamins/Multiminerals have been around for a long time now and a many people take them or at least have them in their cabinet. They are considered by many to be a nutritional "insurance policy" in case you don't eat perfectly and you have a few gaps in your micronutrient nutrition. These micronutrients aren't absorbed as well as micronutrients in their natural state but multivitamins can help you get in the minimal nutrients you need for general health. Some individuals may also more nutrients than the average sedentary person.

Cost: The cost for multivitamins is very minimal. A generic bottle of multivitamins that will last you a year costs about $10, a name brand bottle up to $20. Don't bother with any of those extremely expensive "super-multivitamins" out there that come in packs of 5 or more pills. They contain so many ingredients and such high doses that they just will end up bothering your stomach and wallet. You end up urinating out most of the excess B-vitamins just like you flush away your money with these products. As far as costs, investing in a multivitamin might be one of the most affordable nutritional decisions you can make.

Risks/Side Effects: There are very few possible side effects of taking a multivitamin/multimineral once daily. You do not want to overload your body with fat soluble vitamins such as Vitamin A and E because they can potentially become toxic in large amounts. You also don't want to overload on certain minerals if you are already getting enough throughout the day. Men should try to purchase Iron-Free multivitamins if possible (Men's Multivitamins).

Fish Oil/Flaxseed Oil

General Information: Fish Oil and Flaxseed Oil Capsules are both excellent sources of Omega-3 Fatty Acids. These healthy fats provide several crucial benefits including raising good cholesterol (HDL) and lowering bad cholesterol (LDL). I would recommend taking 1-2 capsules at once, 2-3 times per day to get the full benefits. Both are pretty inexpensive, the flaxseed oil is a little more expensive than the fish oil but I would rather not have the risk of potential mercury contamination. These both contain the extremely beneficial Omega-3 Fatty Acids that can lower bad cholesterol and raise beneficial cholesterol levels. It has also been suggested to help reduce joint inflammation and promote a healthier heart overall. I would suggest taking 1-3 1000g capsules per day on most days when you don't eat fatty fish such as salmon. I've been known to take up to 5 or 6 per day. Make sure the fish oil capsules you are getting are from reputable brands that purify it to remove any toxic mercury (check label). Actual flaxseeds can be crushed and sprinkled on cereal, oatmeal, salads, etc. if you do not want to take capsules. They can also be purchased as ground flaxseed.

Cost: A large container of Fish Oil capsules will cost you about $10 but you can often enjoy a Buy-One-Get-One free deal at CVS or other retailers. A large container of Flax Seed Oil capsules will cost you around $12-15, a little bit more but still worth the price in my opinion.

Risks/Side Effects: No major side effects for Omega-3 capsules except for upset stomachs, diarrhea, and bloating. Omega-3 capsules should not be taken if you are on cholesterol, blood pressure, heart, and some other medications. Avoid Cod Liver Oil as it has a much higher risk of mercury contamination, and it is also sometimes more expensive! If you are purchasing any type of fish oil, make sure it is from a reputable brand so hopefully the risk of mercury contamination is miniscule.

Vitamin C

General Information: Vitamin C is important because it is a powerful antioxidant that can destroy free radicals and help to stimulate the immune system. It is also important for other daily bodily functions and processes. While I do not recommend taking mega-doses of Vitamin C, a capsule or tablet supplement per day or when you are feeling under the weather can help to make a difference. If you are perfectly healthy and consuming enough fruits and vegetables daily, you probably don't need Vitamin C supplements.

Cost: A large bottle of Vitamin C tablets or capsules will run you about $10-15 and last you almost a year even if you took one every day. There are different forms of Vitamin C, Vitamin C with other vitamins, and Vitamin C with herbs such as Rose Hips but I wouldn't pay extra for them.

Risks/Side Effects: There are no major side effects on record for Vitamin C since it is a water soluble vitamin. I would recommend purchasing the bottle with the lowest amount of Vitamin C content, as this will still be 100% or less per serving. Taking 300%, or even 5000% will probably not have any more benefit than taking 100% and you will just end up excreting the rest of the Vitamin C your body did not utilize. If you take enormously large doses of Vitamin C consistently you may risk health problems.

Emergen-C

General Information: Each packet of EmergenC contains massive amounts of Vitamin C in various forms as well as plenty of B-vitamins, electrolytes, and other micronutrients. I find it especially useful for preventing or reducing sickness as well as a good overall addition to your post-workout nutrition. I try to take one in the morning when I wake up and another one post-workout with my protein shake and carbs for its sugar and vitamin content.

Cost: A box of 36 packets costs $10 or less at Wal-Mart. There are also new Immune Defense versions that are slightly more expensive with extra Zinc and antioxidants but the price difference is only a couple dollars per box. I've also found great deals on the CVS generic version where you buy 36 packets for $10 and get another box of 36 for free! Overall, EmergenC and its generic forms are the most affordable and effective option on the market compared to other similar products.

Risks/Side Effects: This product is pretty acidic so may not be ideal for someone with acid reflux disease or a sensitive stomach. Some people may want to avoid this and similar products if they are trying to maintain alkalinity. There are very large amounts of Vitamin C and B Vitamins but they are all water soluble so they will not accumulate in your body and become toxic. It does contain smaller amounts of fat soluble vitamins and minerals which can accumulate in your system. Keep this in mind if you are already taking a multivitamin or other supplements supplying these nutrients.

Calcium + Vitamin D

General Information: The reason I am grouping these two together is because they often come as a combined supplement because they work synergistically. Calcium and Vitamin D are cheap and sometimes necessary supplements, for many women at risk of osteopenia or osteoporosis. There are plenty of reasons to make sure you are taking your daily Vitamin D, or to increase your amounts. First off, since most of us will have minimal exposure to the sun, our natural production of Vitamin D will be very low. This is especially true for those living in colder and darker climates. There are also more cases of Vitamin D deficiency today because of people avoiding sun exposure for fear of melanoma and skin cancer. Vitamin D is crucial for bone health, disease prevention, and optimal calcium absorption. All of us, especially women more susceptible to low bone density, should make sure we get in more dairy products, food fortified with extra Vitamin D, and perhaps even a Calcium + Vitamin D supplement. Low bone density can lead to osteopenia or even osteoporosis and broken bones. If you are unsure of your bone density, see if a bone scan is covered under your insurance.

Cost: A Calcium and Vitamin D generic supplement are very affordable at about $8 for a bottle of 100 tablets. There are various "higher absorption" calcium supplements and different forms of calcium you can take but even these brand name supplements do not cost more than $15 for a bottle. I would recommend you purchase the generic form unless your doctor or registered dietitian says otherwise.

Risks/Side Effects: There are almost no risks of taking a Calcium and Vitamin D supplement as directed. You don't want to take in too much calcium in your diet per day but taking a couple of tablets a day shouldn't put you over the top. Vitamin D is fat soluble but the toxicity level of Vitamin D is very high so that shouldn't be a concern. Check with your pharmacist or physician before adding in a Calcium or Vitamin D supplement.

Whey/Casein Protein Powder

General Information: Protein powder may be one of the most important and versatile supplements out there today. This purified milk protein has very little fat, cholesterol, or carbohydrates and mixes very well in water, juice, or milk. You can even add it to your favorite foods or smoothies. Protein powder helps you to get in your daily required amount of protein in a quick and convenient form that you can take anywhere. Protein powder, whey protein especially, tends to fill people up as well so their appetite for junk food may be reduced. Getting in your protein in an easily digestible liquid form is also ideal post-workout (Chandler et al, 1994). If you are having trouble getting enough protein in your diet through normal foods, or just need a quick snack that won't derail your progress, protein powder is the way to go. Consuming whey protein pre-workout and/or post-workout may improve lean muscle mass and muscle recovery (Tipton et al, 2007). Dymatize Elite 12 Hour Protein is my favorite choice because it is extremely affordable, tastes good, and is high quality. It also has no saturated fat, cholesterol, or sugars. This is the best overall value for protein powder I've had so far.

Cost: Whey and Casein protein powders can vary greatly in price depending on what brand you get, what else they put in there, and the size tub you purchase. I've seen "advanced" 2 lb protein powder tubs for $30-40 and I've seen 4.4 lb tubs for $26 (Dymatize). Opt for the latter. When you do the math out, each scoop ends up being about 50 cents which is very reasonable.

Risks/Side Effects: There are very few reported side effects on protein powder. The only main complaints include stomach discomfort or bloating. Whey protein should only be taken by individuals that have healthy functioning kidneys. You will probably want to opt for soy protein if you are lactose intolerant. Always stay hydrated when taking a protein supplement as this helps to remove the waste by-products of protein metabolism from your system.

Creatine

General Information: Creatine is one of the most proven and researched nutritional supplements on the market. There are many studies demonstrating its ability to improve strength, power, and endurance for both beginners and experts. Other people use it because they think it improves muscle mass and overall weight. Creatine's potential side effect of increasing water retention does not make it an ideal supplement for someone looking to lose or maintain bodyweight. It would only really make sense for strength and power athletes to take, as well as bodybuilders. Do not bother taking creatine if your main objective is to lose weight and tone.

Cost: There are a wide variety of expensive new-age creatine products out there in powder, pill, and even liquid forms. A lot of the newer more advanced creatine is pretty expensive but creatine monohydrate powder is usually pretty cheap. You can get a 2.2 lb tub for about $20 from many vendors, including GNC, possibly less if it's on sale. If you are looking to bulk up, you may also want to look into the Advanced Creatine from Body Fortress which includes a lot of simple sugars, electrolytes, and other nutrients to help with absorption. The Body Fortress Super Advanced Creatine 3 lb tub costs about $16 at Wal-Mart.

Risks/Side Effects: Keep in mind though creatine supplementation is relatively new (less than 20 years of use by the general public) and there are no long-term studies on possible side effects or dangers. Do not take creatine if you are pregnant, nursing, or have kidney/liver problems. Make sure to stay hydrated while taking creatine products as it may increase water retention in the muscle cells. I wouldn't recommend taking more than 5 or 6 grams per day regardless of your size or goals. I have personally been taking creatine on and off for about 7 years and I have never had any problems from it. I have found significant benefits in strength, muscle size, power, and muscular endurance.

Kickers Energy Spray

General Information: Kickers 80 Hour Energy Spray is basically a caffeinated spray that is meant to be used as a sublingual (held under the tongue so it enters the bloodstream quicker). Taking 5 sprays provides you with approximately 200 mg of caffeine, about the same amount as a premium cup of coffee. It also contains large amounts of B-vitamins. Each container has about 80 sprays in it total so that means you get 16 servings for an incredibly low price. While I don't tout this product as "healthy", it is certainly a convenient, affordable, efficient, and very powerful source of caffeine. If you need a quick burst of energy this could be your ticket.

Cost: I've seen bottles priced between $2 and $4 at CVS and Wal-Mart. Either way, this might be the cheapest and most efficient ways to get in your caffeine and B-vitamins. Each small bottle contains 80 sprays so it can last you awhile if you use it in small doses. I don't see it in stores as much these days but you can always purchase it online for a slightly higher price.

Risks/Side Effects: See *A Note on Caffeine* Also contains large amounts of Niacin that can cause flushing of the skin for some, especially in the face. This is supposedly harmless though and I never had any issues related to it. It also tends to go away after using it the first few times as your body gets used to it. A lot of people dislike the flavor and aftertaste because it is very acidic and contains a lot of artificial sweeteners. Because it is so potent, be careful to use as directed and avoid completely if you have caffeine sensitivity, hypertension, or heart disease.

4C Energy Rush Packets

General Information: I first started getting these about 2 years ago when I realized that each packet had the same exact ingredients as two 8 oz Sugar Free Red Bull...but at about 1/8 of the price! They used to have 3 boxes with flavor choices of orange, citrus, or berry with 14 packets in each box. Now they have variety packs with 18 packets in each box for the same price! Each packet mixes in about 16 oz of water (more or less depending on your tastes), tastes excellent, and gives you a big and convenient pick-me-up. If you like energy drinks (especially sugar-free ones) or you are a fellow caffeine-addict, you definitely need to check out this incredible bargain of a product. This product actually makes energy drinks affordable.

Cost: A box of 18 packets (6 Berry, 6 Orange, and 6 Citrus) will cost you between $3.99 and $5.99 depending on where you buy them and if they are on sale. Either way, you are only paying about 25 cents per packet instead of $2-3 for a can of the leading energy drink.

Risks/Side Effects: See "A Note On Caffeine". Also, there are large amounts of artificial sweeteners and acids in this product which may trigger stomach discomfort or headaches in some. These are very potent and should only be used cautiously and as directed.

Caffeine Tablets

General Information: Caffeine is a powerful drug that has stimulant properties that can increase your metabolism, fat burning, and energy while decreasing pain and fatigue. Caffeine is naturally occurring in tea, coffee, chocolate, yerba mate, and other foods. When caffeine is combined with a healthy diet and exercise regimen, it may help to enhance fat loss results. I'm not personally endorsing that anyone start popping caffeine pills, but if you are currently paying $4 for a cup of coffee or an energy drink, you have to realize that the same amount of caffeine is in a 10 cent pill. It puts things in perspective if you are simply looking for a caffeine boost and not necessarily the taste or enjoyment of a cup of coffee, tea, or energy drink.

Cost: A generic container of about 100 caffeine tablets costs about $10 at CVS. Brand name "fat burner" pills are often little more than caffeine and some added herbs and B-Vitamins but they cost about three to five times more.

Risks/Side Effects: See "A Note On Caffeine". Also keep in mind that caffeine is addicting and having a cheap bottle of easily ingested caffeine pills can be very dangerous for some people to have around. This may sound ridiculous but it is a lot easier to overdose on pills than on energy drinks or coffee. If you have a problem with pills or addiction, do not purchase caffeine pills of any type.

A Note On Caffeine

The most common drug in the world is not alcohol, over the counter pain relievers, or tobacco. It is our good friend caffeine and it is warmly embraced by the culture of the United States and the rest of the world. Usually it is in the form of coffee or tea but there are more and more caffeinated concoctions and products on the market every day now (and I've probably tried them all). From my experiences of working 50-60 hour weeks for years at a time, I've learned that when the going gets tough, the tough drink caffeine. It's a necessity for crazy people like me that burn the candle at both ends. But what does caffeine really do to your health? There is a lot of controversy over the pros and cons of coffee and other caffeine-containing products so I'd like to help clear up some misconceptions and state the facts.

Caffeine is a legal drug (except in moderate-large amounts for NCAA and Olympic athletes) with stimulant properties that increase the heart rate, increase metabolism, and create diuretic effects. Caffeine intake helps burn significantly larger amounts of fat for energy, which makes it the key ingredient in nearly all weight loss pills and diets on the market. It can also increase feelings of happiness, mental alertness, energy levels, and cardiovascular endurance. Moderate to high levels of caffeine correlates with a reduced risk in Parkinson's Disease, heart disease, and many other serious conditions. Caffeine can even temporarily relieve pain and is included in many headache and migraine medications. It truly is a wonder drug if taken correctly, but chronically large intakes can lead to some major health problems in many individuals.

Like any other drug, caffeine can be very addicting. In fact, the major reason why soft drink companies originally added it to their drinks was to create addiction to their product. I'm sure if it were possible (and maybe it will be at some point), big tobacco would have added caffeine to cigarettes to add to the already potent addictive properties of nicotine. If you stop consuming caffeine after consistently high usage, your body will start to go through a variety of withdrawal symptoms. You can have mood changes due to hormonal and other chemical imbalances in your brain. Without caffeine many people feel lethargic, may have severe headaches, and can feel nauseous. These symptoms subside in days or weeks but they can be extremely debilitating in certain individuals, especially when mixed with other drugs or alcohol. Also remember that taking caffeine can dehydrate you so you'll need to drink a lot of extra water throughout the day. Most health and fitness professionals will advocate drinking an 8 oz glass of water for every 8 oz cup of tea or coffee consumed. For most, caffeine shouldn't be taken at night or sleep disturbances or disorders will occur.

Although I don't always follow my own advice, I would recommend 1-2 8 oz cups of coffee (or up to 3 cups of caffeinated tea) per day at the most to gain its benefits and minimize any potential health issues. Abstain from caffeine completely once or twice a week so you do not continue to build an even greater tolerance to it. If you do drink large amounts of caffeine temporarily, try to wean off it slowly over a period of several days or a week. Enjoy your caffeine but please drink or supplement with it in moderation. As always, check with your physician, pharmacist, and/or registered dietitian to make sure you are healthy enough to consume caffeine and that it won't interact negatively with any of your medications. Bottoms up!

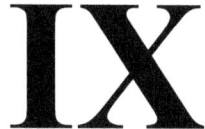

IX

Works Cited

Academic Journals:

- Almada, Anthony L., B. Kreider, Conrad P. Earnest, Jennifer Lundberg, Christopher Rasmussen, Michael Greenwood, and Patricia Cowan. Effects of ingesting protein with various forms of carbohydrate following resistance-exercise on substrate availability and markers of anabolism, catabolism, and immunity. *J Int Soc Sports Nutr* 4.18 (Nov 12, 2007): p18

- Campbell B, Kreider RB, Ziegenfuss T, La Bounty P, Roberts M, Burke D, Landis J, Lopez H, Antonio J: International Society of Sports Nutrition Position Stand: Protein and Exercise. *J Int Soc Sports Nutr* 2007, 4(1): 8.

- Chandler RM, Byrne HK, Patterson JG, Ivy JL: Dietary supplements affect the anabolic hormones after weight-training exercise. *J Appl Physiol* 1994, 76(2): 839-845.

- Conley MS, Stone MH: Carbohydrate ingestion/supplementation or resistance exercise and training. *Sports Med* 1996, 21(1): 7-17.

- Kraemer WJ, Volek JS, Bush JA, Putukian M, Sebastianelli WJ: Hormonal responses to consecutive days of heavy-resistance exercise with or without nutritional supplementation. *J Appl Physiol* 1998, 85(4): 1544-1555.

- Tipton KD, Elliott TA, Cree MG, Aarsland AA, Sanford AP, Wolfe RR: Stimulation of net muscle protein synthesis by whey protein ingestion before and after exercise. *Am J Physiol Endocrinol Metab* 2007, 292(1): E71-76.

- Karstadt, Myra L. Testing needed for acesulfame potassium, an artificial sweetener. (Correspondence). *Journal of Environmental Health Perspectives.* 114.9 (Sept 2006): pA516(1).

- Migraine Triggered by Sucralose-A Case Report. *Headache: Journal of Head and Face Pain.* 47.3 (March 2007): p447(1).

- Szalavltz, Maia. The sweetener standoff: Maia Szalavltz weighs in on the controversy involving artificial sweetners. *Psychology Today.* 39.5 (Sept-Oct 2006): p60(1)

- Vessby B, Unsitupa M, Hermansen K, Riccardi G, Rivellese AA, Tapsell LC, Nälsén C, Berglund L, Louheranta A, Rasmussen BM, Calvert GD, Maffetone A, Pedersen E, Gustafsson IB, Storlien LH (2001)."Substituting dietary saturated for monounsaturated fat impairs insulin sensitivity in healthy men and women: The KANWU Study". *Diabetologia* 44 (3): 312 9. doi:10.1007/s001250051620.PMID 11317662.

Books:
- Hatfield, F. 2004. Fitness: The Complete Guide, Official Text for ISSA's Certified Fitness Trainer Program. International Sports Science Association.

Websites:

- www.bmi-calculator.net

The Frugal Workout

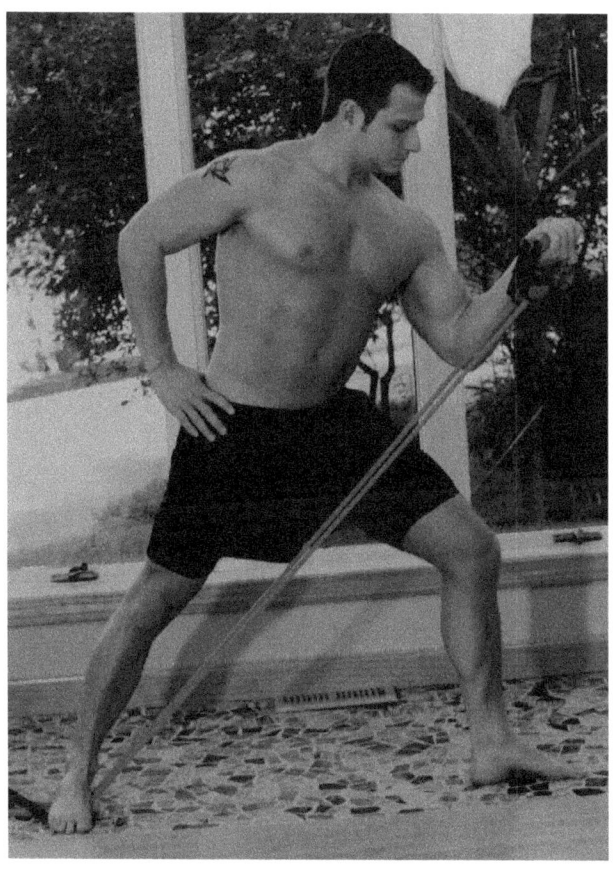

Are You Taking The Frugal Diet Challenge? Do you want to take your workouts to the next level without spending a fortune on gym memberships, personal trainers, or fitness equipment? Download your copy of the Best-Selling E-Book "The Frugal Workout" today and get even better results. Coming out in paperback in 2011!

About The Author

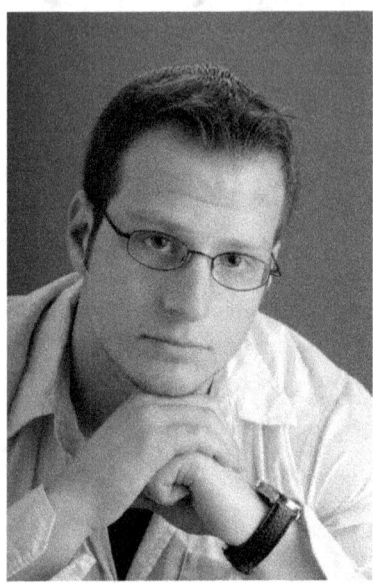

Author Michael J. Schiemer has been a Personal Trainer for 8 years and has worked in all areas of the fitness industry. He is the proud owner of RESULTS Private Fitness, Greater Boston's premier in-home and online personal training and nutrition company. He graduated with honors from Merrimack College with a Bachelor's of Science in Sports Medicine and a Concentration in Exercise Physiology. He holds a dozen nationally recognized fitness certifications and is a member of the National Strength and Conditioning Association. Michael has helped hundreds of clients improve their health and fitness levels through proper exercise, nutrition, and lifestyle advice. He has competed in natural bodybuilding and powerlifting and has always promoted a drug-free approach to fitness, sports, and weight training. He has also worked as a fitness model, life coach, health club manager, and marketing consultant. He has worked with everyone including professional athletes, youth athletes, CEOs, models, doctors, and special needs clients. Michael also enjoys marketing, technology, business development, sports, heavy metal, and animals. He lives in Boston, MA with his cat Chewie and dog Dudley.

Michael J. Schiemer Wants To Connect With You!

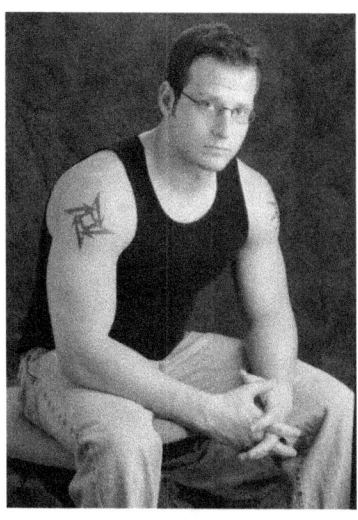

Michael is online and would love to hear your feedback on the book and discuss all things health and fitness. Connect with him on his personal, business, and social media sites!

RESULTS Private Fitness:
www.resultsprivatefitness.com
YouTube Fitness Channel:
www.youtube.com/mikeschiemercpt
Facebook Fan Page:
www.facebook.com/mikeschiemer
Twitter:
www.twitter.com/mikeschiemer
Fitness Blog:
www.mikeschiemer.blogspot.com
LinkedIn:
www.linkedin.com/in/mikeschiemer

Become a Fan of The Frugal Diet on Facebook!
Discuss Your Success Stories With Other Readers!
http://facebook.com/thefrugaldiet

The Frugal Diet Team:

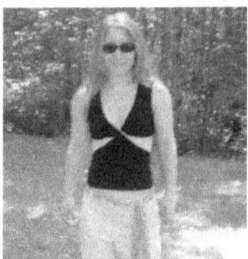

Chef Corin Szostek

Corin is an award-winning chef living in Rehoboth, MA. She works in the food service industry and is an up-and-coming fitness /nutritional consultant.

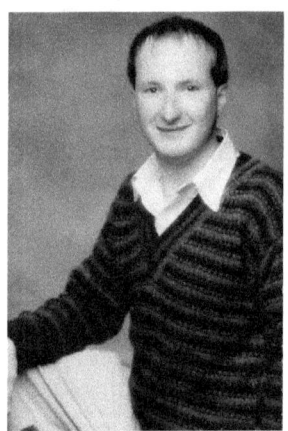

Chef Mark Brambilla
www.culinaryadventuresathome.webs.com

Mark has been an award-winning chef for nearly two decades and has served thousands of satisfied clients and customers of all types. Mark is the graduate of Johnson and Whales University for food management as well as USPCI for medical nutrition. He also specializes in catering, organic cooking, and macrobiotic cooking. Mark also specializes in saving his clients money while improving their level of nutrition. He is the owner of Culinary Adventures At Home and he resides in Walpole, MA.

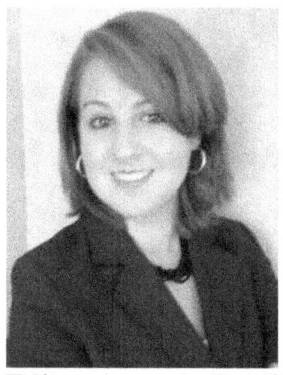

Editor Amanda Baldi
www.amandabaldi.com
www.abaldi.blogspot.com

Amanda is an award-winning independent writer and editor. She graduated with honors with a Degrees in both English and Comparative Literature. She is also a talented artist and cook that studied abroad in Italy. She is the owner of In Bold By Baldi and resides in Walpole, MA.

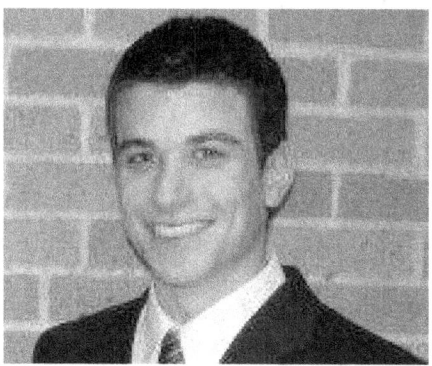

Photographer David A. Schiemer

David is a dean's list and scholarship engineering student at Lehigh University and a rising entrepreneur. He excels in many areas including photography, sports, fitness, writing, painting, landscaping, construction, and E-Commerce. He currently resides in Medfield, MA.

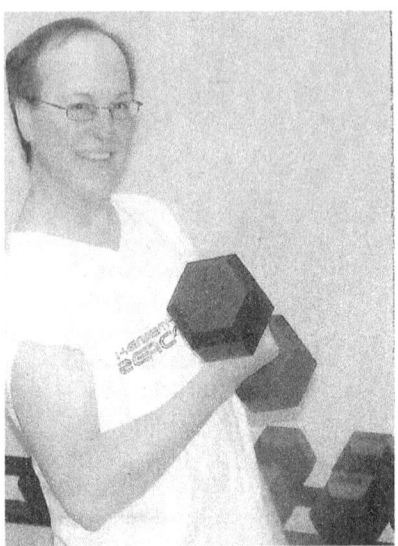

Photographer Robert Thomson

Robert Thomson, a former personal training client of mine, has been active in the hair and beauty industry for decades as a highly sought-after hair stylist and make-up artist. He has owned his own beauty salon and a successful cosmetics product company. He is growing his credentials as a modeling photographer and graphic designer.

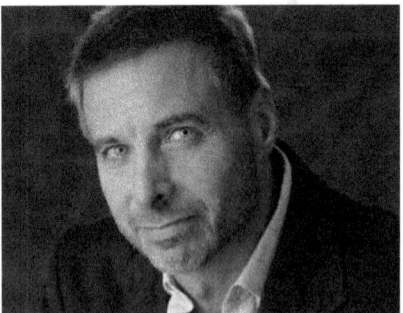

Photographer Peter Swiniarski

Peter has been a photographer for over 20 years as well as a personal trainer. He is a 5-time Pan Mass Challenge cycling veteran and is a strong advocate for The Jimmy Fund and Dana Farber Cancer Research institute. He resides in Methuen, MA.

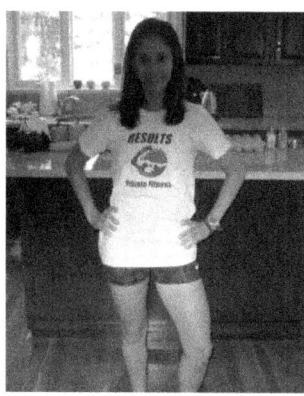

Cover Model Julie Zaia
www.dystonia-foundation.org

Julie is a Registered Dietitian and 5-time marathon runner. She has a bachelor's degree in nutritional science from Clemson University and has been Certified as a Personal Trainer and Nutrition Specialist. She is a very strong advocate for the Dystonia Foundation. She currently resides in Atlanta, GA.

My Other Recipe Contributors

Contributor   **Organization/Website**
- Lisa Gardiner
- Nancy Schiemer
- Marissa Bognanno   adventuresintheboot.blogspot.com
- Paige Clunie   www.826boston.org
- Worcester Earn a Bike   www.worcesterearnabike.org
- Sue Lasch
- Joanne Koch
- Luanne Monahan
- Crissy Kreuger
- Mirella Santucci   JGS Enterprises of Medfield, Inc
- Catherine Lawrie
- Paula Pelavin   Sick of the Bull
- Kate Koch
- Nicholas Sullivan   www.ajunkyard.wordpress.com
- Lori Cushner
- Heather Mayer
- Sarah Klein
- Christine Van Zadelhoff

Get
RESULTS

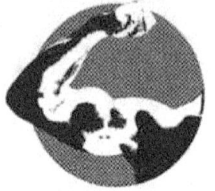

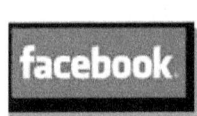

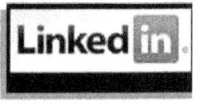

www.resultsprivatefitness.com

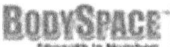   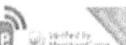

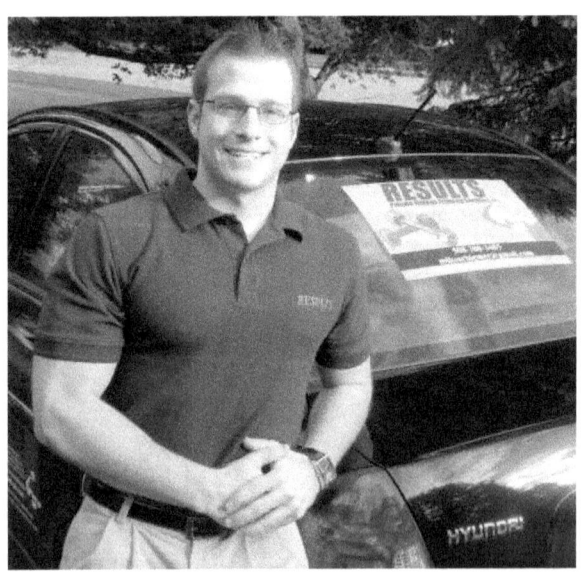

"Invest In Your Health"